The Easy Guide To 2000-Days Of Low-Sugar, Low-Carb Diabetic Friendly Recipes For Newly Diagnosed With A 31-Day Meal Plan To Control Blood Sugar

Marcus Baron

Table of Contents

COPYRIGHT © 2023

CHAPTER ONE

Understanding Diabetes and Low Carb Nutrition

Introduction to Diabetes and its Relationship with Carbohydrates

Diabetes is a chronic metabolic disorder characterized by high blood sugar levels over a prolonged period. This condition arises due to the body's inability to produce enough insulin or effectively utilize the insulin it produces. Insulin is a hormone produced by the pancreas that helps regulate blood sugar levels by facilitating the uptake of glucose from the bloodstream into cells for energy or storage.

There are two main types of diabetes: type 1 and type 2.

Type 1 Diabetes: Type 1 diabetes is an autoimmune condition where the immune system attacks and destroys insulin-producing beta cells in the pancreas. This results in little to no insulin production, requiring individuals with type 1 diabetes to rely on insulin injections for survival.

Type 2 Diabetes: Type 2 diabetes, on the other hand, is characterized by insulin resistance, where cells become less responsive to insulin's action, leading to elevated blood sugar levels. Initially, the pancreas compensates by producing more insulin, but over time, it may fail to keep up with the body's demands, resulting in high blood sugar levels.

Carbohydrates play a significant role in blood sugar management because they are broken down into glucose, which enters the bloodstream and raises blood sugar levels. Therefore, carbohydrate intake is a crucial consideration for individuals with diabetes, as it directly impacts their blood sugar levels.

Benefits of a Low Carb Diet for Diabetics

A low carb diet restricts the intake of carbohydrates, thereby reducing the amount of glucose entering the bloodstream. This can offer several benefits for individuals with diabetes:

1. **Improved Blood Sugar Control:** By reducing carbohydrate intake, a low carb diet can help stabilize blood sugar levels, reducing the risk of hyperglycemia (high blood sugar) and hypoglycemia (low blood sugar). This can lead to better overall glycemic control, which is essential for managing diabetes and preventing complications.

2. **Weight Management:** Low carb diets have been shown to be effective for weight loss and weight maintenance. Excess body weight is a significant risk factor for type 2 diabetes and can exacerbate insulin resistance. By promoting weight loss, a low carb diet can improve insulin sensitivity and help manage diabetes more effectively.

3. **Reduced Dependency on Medications:** Some individuals with diabetes may be able to reduce their reliance on medications, including insulin and oral hypoglycemic agents, by following a low carb diet. By stabilizing blood sugar levels through dietary modifications, it may be possible to lower medication doses or even eliminate the need for certain medications under medical supervision.

4. **Improved Lipid Profile:** Low carb diets have been associated with improvements in lipid profile, including reductions in triglycerides and increases in HDL (good) cholesterol levels. These changes can reduce the risk of cardiovascular disease, which is a significant concern for individuals with diabetes.

5. **Increased Satiety:** Low carb diets often include foods that are rich in protein and healthy fats, which can increase feelings of fullness and satiety. This can help individuals with diabetes control their appetite and reduce cravings for high-carbohydrate foods, making it easier to adhere to their dietary plan.

6. **Better Insulin Sensitivity:** Restricting carbohydrate intake can improve insulin sensitivity, allowing cells to more effectively respond to insulin's action and lowering blood sugar levels. This can be particularly beneficial for individuals with type 2 diabetes, where insulin resistance is a key underlying factor.

Basic Principles of Low Carb Eating for Diabetes Management

Adopting a low carb diet for diabetes management involves several key principles:

1. **Limit Carbohydrate Intake:** The primary focus of a low carb diet is to restrict carbohydrate intake, typically to around 20-50 grams of net carbs per day. Net carbs are calculated by subtracting fiber from total carbohydrates since fiber does not significantly impact blood sugar levels.

2. **Choose Nutrient-Dense Foods:** While reducing carbs, it's essential to prioritize nutrient-dense foods that provide essential vitamins, minerals, and antioxidants. This includes non-starchy vegetables, lean proteins, healthy fats, and moderate amounts of low glycemic index fruits.

3. **Emphasize Whole Foods:** Processed and refined carbohydrates should be minimized or avoided, as they can cause rapid spikes in blood sugar levels. Instead, focus on whole foods that are minimally processed and rich in fiber, such as whole grains, nuts, seeds, and legumes.

4. **Monitor Blood Sugar Levels:** Regular monitoring of blood sugar levels is essential for individuals with diabetes, especially when making dietary changes. This allows for adjustments to carbohydrate intake based on individual

blood sugar responses and helps ensure optimal glycemic control.

5. **Stay Hydrated:** Adequate hydration is crucial for overall health and can help prevent complications associated with diabetes. Water is the best choice for hydration, but herbal teas and sugar-free beverages can also be included.

6. **Consult a Healthcare Professional:** Before making significant changes to your diet, especially if you have diabetes, it's important to consult with a healthcare professional or registered dietitian. They can provide personalized guidance based on your medical history, dietary preferences, and health goals.

In conclusion, a low carb diet can be a valuable tool for managing diabetes and improving overall health outcomes. By reducing carbohydrate intake, individuals with diabetes can achieve better blood sugar control, promote weight loss, and reduce the risk of complications associated with the condition. However, it's essential to approach low carb eating with a focus on nutrient density, whole foods, and personalized guidance from healthcare professionals.

CHAPTER TWO

Essential Tools and Ingredients for Low Carb Cooking

Stocking Your Kitchen with Low Carb Staples

Creating a well-equipped kitchen is essential for successful low carb cooking. Here's a list of low carb staples to keep on hand:

1. **Non-Starchy Vegetables:** Fill your fridge with low carb vegetables such as spinach, kale, broccoli, cauliflower, zucchini, bell peppers, and mushrooms. These veggies are versatile and can be used in a variety of dishes, from salads to stir-fries.

2. **Protein Sources:** Stock up on lean proteins like chicken breast, turkey, fish, tofu, and eggs. Protein is essential for building and repairing tissues and can help you feel full and satisfied after meals.

3. **Healthy Fats:** Include sources of healthy fats in your pantry, such as olive oil, avocado oil, coconut oil, and nuts/seeds. These fats provide energy, support cell growth, and help absorb fat-soluble vitamins.

4. **Low Carb Flours and Baking Ingredients:** Almond flour, coconut flour, and flaxseed meal are excellent alternatives to traditional wheat flour for low carb baking. Other baking

essentials include baking powder, baking soda, and sugar-free sweeteners.

5. **Sugar-Free Condiments and Sauces:** Look for sugar-free versions of condiments like mustard, mayonnaise, hot sauce, and soy sauce to add flavor to your dishes without the added carbs.

6. **Herbs and Spices:** Build a collection of herbs and spices to add flavor to your meals without adding extra calories or carbs. Some popular options include garlic powder, onion powder, cumin, paprika, and Italian seasoning.

7. **Nuts and Seeds:** Keep a variety of nuts and seeds on hand for snacking or adding crunch to your dishes. Options like almonds, walnuts, chia seeds, and sunflower seeds are low in carbs and high in healthy fats and fiber.

8. **Low Carb Pasta and Rice Alternatives:** Explore alternatives to traditional pasta and rice, such as spiralized zucchini (zoodles), spaghetti squash, shirataki noodles, and cauliflower rice. These options allow you to enjoy your favorite dishes while keeping carb counts low.

9. **Sugar-Free Snacks:** Keep a selection of sugar-free snacks on hand for when cravings strike. Options like cheese sticks, beef jerky, pork rinds, and sugar-free jello can satisfy hunger without derailing your low carb diet.

10.   **Low Carb Dairy Products:** Choose dairy products that are low in carbs, such as unsweetened almond milk, coconut milk, Greek yogurt, and cheese. These dairy options provide calcium and protein without the added sugars found in some dairy products.

By stocking your kitchen with these low carb staples, you'll have everything you need to prepare delicious and satisfying meals while sticking to your dietary goals.

Must-Have Kitchen Equipment for Low Carb Meal Preparation

Having the right kitchen equipment can make low carb meal preparation easier and more enjoyable. Here are some essential tools to have on hand:

1. **High-Quality Chef's Knife:** A sharp chef's knife is essential for chopping vegetables, slicing meats, and other food preparation tasks. Invest in a high-quality knife that feels comfortable and balanced in your hand.

2. **Cutting Board:** Choose a durable cutting board made from wood or plastic that won't dull your knives. Having a separate cutting board for meat and vegetables can help prevent cross-contamination.

3. **Vegetable Spiralizer:** A vegetable spiralizer is a handy tool for creating low carb pasta alternatives like zoodles (zucchini

noodles) or spiralized carrots. Look for a spiralizer with multiple blade options for versatility.

4. **Food Processor or Blender:** A food processor or blender is useful for making sauces, dressings, and smoothies. It can also be used to chop nuts, blend cauliflower into rice-like grains, or puree vegetables for soups and sauces.

5. **Cast Iron Skillet or Non-Stick Pan:** A cast iron skillet or non-stick pan is essential for cooking meats, sautéing vegetables, and making omelets or frittatas. These pans distribute heat evenly and require less oil for cooking.

6. **Baking Sheets and Pans:** Stock your kitchen with baking sheets and pans for roasting vegetables, baking low carb desserts, and making sheet pan meals. Opt for non-stick or silicone-coated options for easy cleanup.

7. **Slow Cooker or Instant Pot:** A slow cooker or Instant Pot can be a lifesaver for busy weeknights. Use it to prepare low carb soups, stews, and casseroles with minimal effort.

8. **Measuring Cups and Spoons:** Accurate measurement is crucial for low carb baking and cooking. Invest in a set of measuring cups and spoons to ensure consistent results.

9. **Kitchen Scale:** A kitchen scale is handy for measuring ingredients by weight, especially for baking recipes that

require precise measurements. It's also useful for portion control and tracking macros.

10. **Silicone Baking Mats and Parchment Paper:** Silicone baking mats and parchment paper are essential for lining baking sheets and pans, preventing food from sticking and making cleanup a breeze.

By outfitting your kitchen with these essential tools, you'll be well-equipped to tackle any low carb recipe with confidence and ease.

Understanding Low Carb Sweeteners and Alternatives

When following a low carb diet, finding suitable alternatives to sugar is essential for satisfying your sweet tooth without spiking blood sugar levels. Here's a guide to understanding low carb sweeteners and alternatives:

1. **Stevia:** Stevia is a natural sweetener derived from the leaves of the Stevia rebaudiana plant. It's calorie-free and much sweeter than sugar, so only a small amount is needed to sweeten foods and beverages. Stevia is available in liquid, powder, and granulated forms and can be used in cooking and baking.

2. **Erythritol:** Erythritol is a sugar alcohol that occurs naturally in some fruits and fermented foods. It's virtually calorie-free and doesn't raise blood sugar levels, making it an excellent

option for low carb diets. Erythritol has a similar taste and texture to sugar and can be used in baking, cooking, and sweetening beverages.

3. **Monk Fruit Sweetener:** Monk fruit sweetener is made from extracts of the monk fruit, a small green gourd native to Southeast Asia. Like stevia, monk fruit sweetener is calorie-free and much sweeter than sugar. It's available in granulated and powdered forms and can be used as a sugar substitute in various recipes.

4. **Xylitol:** Xylitol is another sugar alcohol commonly used as a low carb sweetener. It has fewer calories than sugar and a low glycemic index, making it suitable for individuals with diabetes. Xylitol has a similar taste and sweetness to sugar and can be used in baking, cooking, and sweetening beverages.

5. **Allulose:** Allulose is a rare sugar found naturally in small quantities in certain foods like wheat, figs, and raisins. It has minimal impact on blood sugar levels and provides about 70% of the sweetness of sugar with fewer calories. Allulose behaves similarly to sugar in recipes and can be used in baking, cooking, and sweetening beverages.

6. **Sugar Alcohols:** In addition to erythritol and xylitol, other sugar alcohols like sorbitol and maltitol are commonly used as low carb sweeteners. While they provide fewer calories

and have a lower glycemic index than sugar, some people may experience digestive issues like gas and bloating when consuming large amounts of sugar alcohols.

7. **Artificial Sweeteners:** Artificial sweeteners like aspartame (Equal), sucralose (Splenda), and saccharin (Sweet'N Low) are calorie-free and intensely sweet, making them popular choices for low carb diets. However, some artificial sweeteners may have a bitter aftertaste or raise concerns about long-term health effects, so use them in moderation.

When choosing low carb sweeteners, consider factors like taste, sweetness level, and potential side effects. Experiment with different options to find the ones that work best for your taste preferences and dietary needs. Keep in mind that while low carb sweeteners can be useful for reducing sugar intake, they should still be consumed in moderation as part of a balanced diet.

CHAPTER THREE

Breakfasts to Start Your Day Right

Quick and Delicious Low Carb Breakfast Ideas

Starting your day with a nutritious breakfast sets the tone for healthy eating habits and provides you with the energy you need to tackle the day ahead. Here are some quick and delicious low carb breakfast ideas to kickstart your morning:

1. **Egg Muffins:** Whip up a batch of egg muffins by whisking together eggs, diced vegetables, cheese, and your choice of protein (such as cooked bacon or sausage). Pour the mixture into greased muffin tins and bake until set. These portable breakfast bites can be made ahead of time and reheated for a quick morning meal.

2. **Avocado Toast:** Swap traditional toast for sliced avocado as the base of your breakfast. Top with sliced tomatoes, a sprinkle of feta cheese, and a drizzle of olive oil for a satisfying and low carb alternative.

3. **Greek Yogurt Parfait:** Layer Greek yogurt with low carb berries (such as strawberries, raspberries, or blueberries) and a handful of nuts or seeds for added crunch. You can also sweeten the yogurt with a dash of vanilla extract and a sprinkle of stevia or monk fruit sweetener.

4. **Chia Seed Pudding:** Mix chia seeds with unsweetened almond milk or coconut milk and let sit overnight in the fridge. In the morning, top the pudding with sliced almonds, coconut flakes, and a few berries for a nutritious and filling breakfast.

5. **Smoked Salmon Roll-Ups:** Spread cream cheese on slices of smoked salmon and top with sliced cucumber, avocado, and a sprinkle of everything bagel seasoning. Roll up the salmon slices and enjoy these flavorful and protein-packed roll-ups.

6. **Low Carb Breakfast Burrito:** Fill a low carb tortilla or lettuce wrap with scrambled eggs, sautéed vegetables, cheese, and your choice of protein (such as diced ham or turkey sausage). Roll up the burrito and enjoy it hot or cold.

7. **Coconut Flour Pancakes:** Make fluffy pancakes using coconut flour, eggs, almond milk, and a pinch of baking powder. Serve with a dollop of Greek yogurt and fresh berries for a satisfying and low carb breakfast treat.

8. **Cottage Cheese Bowl:** Top cottage cheese with sliced avocado, cherry tomatoes, cucumber slices, and a sprinkle of hemp seeds or sunflower seeds for a quick and protein-rich breakfast option.

9. **Breakfast Salad:** Start your day with a refreshing breakfast salad made with mixed greens, diced avocado, hard-boiled

eggs, crispy bacon bits, and a drizzle of balsamic vinaigrette. This savory salad is a flavorful way to incorporate vegetables into your morning routine.

10.   **Keto Smoothie:** Blend together unsweetened almond milk, spinach, avocado, protein powder, and a handful of low carb berries for a creamy and nutritious keto smoothie. Customize the smoothie with your favorite low carb ingredients, such as chia seeds, flaxseeds, or nut butter, for added flavor and texture.

These quick and delicious low carb breakfast ideas are perfect for busy mornings when you need a nutritious meal on the go. Experiment with different ingredients and flavors to find the combinations that you enjoy most.

High Protein Breakfasts to Keep You Satisfied

A high protein breakfast not only helps keep you feeling full and satisfied until your next meal but also supports muscle repair and growth. Here are some high protein breakfast ideas to fuel your day:

1. **Spinach and Feta Omelet:** Whip up a fluffy omelet filled with sautéed spinach, diced tomatoes, and crumbled feta cheese. Eggs are an excellent source of protein, while spinach adds fiber and vitamins to your meal.

2. **Greek Yogurt Bowl:** Start your day with a bowl of Greek yogurt topped with sliced almonds, chia seeds, and a drizzle of honey or sugar-free syrup. Greek yogurt is rich in protein and probiotics, which support digestive health.

3. **Protein-Packed Smoothie:** Blend together protein powder, unsweetened almond milk, spinach, and frozen berries for a satisfying and nutrient-dense smoothie. You can also add nut butter or Greek yogurt for an extra protein boost.

4. **Turkey and Cheese Roll-Ups:** Roll slices of deli turkey or chicken breast around string cheese or sliced avocado for a quick and portable breakfast option. This protein-packed snack will keep you feeling full and energized throughout the morning.

5. **Smoked Salmon Breakfast Bowl:** Build a breakfast bowl with smoked salmon, sliced avocado, hard-boiled eggs, and cherry tomatoes. Sprinkle with everything bagel seasoning and a squeeze of lemon juice for a flavorful and protein-rich meal.

6. **Quinoa Breakfast Porridge:** Cook quinoa in unsweetened almond milk or coconut milk and top with sliced almonds, chopped dates, and a sprinkle of cinnamon for a hearty and protein-packed breakfast porridge.

7. **Protein Pancakes:** Make pancakes using protein powder, eggs, and mashed bananas for a high protein and low carb

breakfast option. Top with Greek yogurt and fresh berries for added protein and flavor.

8. **Egg and Veggie Breakfast Wrap:** Fill a low carb tortilla or lettuce wrap with scrambled eggs, sautéed vegetables, and shredded cheese for a protein-packed breakfast wrap. This portable meal is perfect for busy mornings on the go.

9. **Cottage Cheese Pancakes:** Mix cottage cheese with eggs, almond flour, and a splash of vanilla extract to make fluffy and protein-rich pancakes. Serve with a dollop of Greek yogurt and sliced strawberries for a delicious and filling breakfast.

10. **Baked Egg Muffins:** Bake eggs in muffin tins with diced vegetables, cheese, and cooked bacon or sausage for a grab-and-go breakfast option. These protein-packed egg muffins can be made ahead of time and reheated throughout the week.

Incorporating high protein breakfasts into your morning routine can help keep you feeling full, satisfied, and energized until your next meal. Experiment with different ingredients and flavors to create delicious and nutritious breakfast options that you enjoy.

Low Carb Smoothies and Breakfast Casseroles

Smoothies and breakfast casseroles are convenient options for busy mornings when you need a quick and satisfying meal. Here are some low carb recipes to try:

Low Carb Smoothies:

1. **Green Protein Smoothie:** Blend together spinach, kale, avocado, protein powder, and unsweetened almond milk for a refreshing and nutrient-dense green smoothie. Add a handful of berries for natural sweetness and antioxidants.

2. **Chocolate Peanut Butter Smoothie:** Combine unsweetened cocoa powder, peanut butter, protein powder, and a frozen banana with unsweetened almond milk for a decadent and protein-rich smoothie. Adjust the sweetness to taste with a dash of stevia or monk fruit sweetener.

3. **Berry Blast Smoothie:** Blend together mixed berries, Greek yogurt, protein powder, and coconut water for a delicious and antioxidant-rich smoothie. Customize the smoothie with your favorite low carb fruits, such as strawberries, blueberries, and raspberries.

4. **Mocha Protein Shake:** Mix brewed coffee, chocolate protein powder, almond milk, and a tablespoon of almond butter for a creamy and satisfying mocha protein shake. Add a sprinkle of cinnamon or cocoa powder for extra flavor.

5. **Tropical Green Smoothie:** Combine spinach, pineapple, mango, protein powder, and coconut water for a tropical-inspired green smoothie. Garnish with shredded coconut and a squeeze of lime juice for a refreshing and nutrient-packed breakfast.

Low Carb Breakfast Casseroles:

1. **Spinach and Feta Breakfast Casserole:** Layer sautéed spinach, crumbled feta cheese, and diced tomatoes in a baking dish. Pour beaten eggs over the top and bake until set for a savory and protein-rich breakfast casserole.

2. **Sausage and Mushroom Breakfast Bake:** Cook crumbled breakfast sausage with sliced mushrooms and onions until browned. Spread the mixture in a baking dish and top with beaten eggs and shredded cheese. Bake until golden and bubbly for a hearty and satisfying breakfast bake.

3. **Ham and Cheese Breakfast Strata:** Layer sliced ham, shredded cheese, and diced bell peppers in a baking dish. Pour beaten eggs mixed with unsweetened almond milk over the top and let sit overnight in the fridge. Bake in the morning until set for a flavorful and protein-packed breakfast strata.

4. **Vegetable Egg Bake:** Sauté diced vegetables such as bell peppers, onions, and zucchini until tender. Spread the

vegetables in a baking dish and top with beaten eggs mixed with shredded cheese. Bake until golden and puffed for a nutritious and satisfying breakfast bake.

5. **Broccoli and Bacon Frittata:** Cook diced bacon until crispy and set aside. Sauté broccoli florets in the bacon drippings until tender. Spread the broccoli and bacon in a baking dish and pour beaten eggs over the top. Bake until set and golden for a flavorful and protein-rich frittata.

Smoothies and breakfast casseroles are versatile options for low carb breakfasts that can be customized with your favorite ingredients and flavors. Whether you prefer a creamy and nutrient-packed smoothie or a hearty and protein-rich casserole, these recipes are sure to start your day off right.

CHAPTER FOUR

Low Carb Lunches for On-the-Go

Easy Salad and Wrap Recipes for Low Carb Lunches

When you're on the go, quick and convenient meals are essential. Here are some easy salad and wrap recipes that are low in carbs and perfect for packed lunches:

Salad Recipes:

1. **Greek Salad:** Toss together chopped cucumbers, tomatoes, red onions, Kalamata olives, and feta cheese with a drizzle of olive oil and lemon juice. Add grilled chicken or shrimp for extra protein, and enjoy this refreshing and flavorful salad on the go.

2. **Cobb Salad:** Arrange chopped romaine lettuce in a container and top with diced avocado, hard-boiled eggs, crispy bacon bits, cherry tomatoes, and crumbled blue cheese. Pack the salad with a side of ranch dressing or vinaigrette for a satisfying and protein-packed lunch.

3. **Caprese Salad:** Layer sliced tomatoes, fresh mozzarella cheese, and basil leaves in a container and drizzle with

balsamic glaze and olive oil. Add a sprinkle of salt and pepper for seasoning, and enjoy this classic Italian salad on the go.

4. **Asian Chicken Salad:** Combine shredded cabbage, carrots, bell peppers, and sliced cucumbers with cooked shredded chicken and chopped peanuts. Toss with a homemade Asian-inspired dressing made from soy sauce, sesame oil, rice vinegar, and ginger for a flavorful and crunchy salad option.

5. **Tuna Salad Lettuce Wraps:** Mix canned tuna with mayonnaise, diced celery, red onion, and lemon juice. Spoon the tuna salad onto large lettuce leaves and roll up to create low carb wraps. Pack the wraps with a side of sliced vegetables or almonds for a satisfying and portable lunch option.

Wrap Recipes:

1. **Turkey and Avocado Wrap:** Spread mashed avocado on a low carb tortilla and top with sliced turkey breast, lettuce, tomato, and bacon. Roll up the tortilla and slice into pinwheels for a delicious and protein-packed wrap.

2. **Mediterranean Veggie Wrap:** Fill a low carb wrap with hummus, roasted vegetables (such as bell peppers, zucchini, and eggplant), feta cheese, and fresh spinach. Roll up the wrap and secure with toothpicks for a flavorful and satisfying lunch option.

3. **Buffalo Chicken Wrap:** Toss cooked shredded chicken with buffalo sauce and Greek yogurt or ranch dressing. Spread the chicken mixture onto a low carb tortilla and top with shredded lettuce, diced tomatoes, and crumbled blue cheese. Roll up the wrap and enjoy this spicy and protein-rich lunch option.

4. **Egg Salad Wrap:** Mix hard-boiled eggs with mayonnaise, mustard, diced celery, and green onions. Spread the egg salad onto a low carb tortilla and top with lettuce leaves and sliced avocado. Roll up the tortilla and slice into pinwheels for a classic and satisfying lunch option.

5. **BLT Lettuce Wraps:** Fill large lettuce leaves with crispy bacon strips, sliced tomatoes, and avocado slices. Drizzle with mayonnaise and roll up the lettuce leaves to create low carb BLT wraps. Pack the wraps with a side of carrot sticks or cucumber slices for a crunchy and satisfying lunch option.

These easy salad and wrap recipes are perfect for on-the-go lunches and can be customized with your favorite ingredients and flavors. Whether you prefer a refreshing salad or a hearty wrap, these low carb options are sure to keep you satisfied throughout the day.

Protein-Packed Lunches to Maintain Energy Levels

Protein is essential for maintaining energy levels and keeping you feeling full and satisfied throughout the day. Here are some protein-packed lunch ideas that are perfect for on-the-go:

1. **Grilled Chicken Salad:** Toss together mixed greens, cherry tomatoes, cucumber slices, and grilled chicken breast strips. Drizzle with balsamic vinaigrette or your favorite dressing for a simple yet satisfying protein-packed salad.

2. **Quinoa and Black Bean Bowl:** Combine cooked quinoa with black beans, diced bell peppers, corn kernels, and shredded cheese. Top with grilled chicken or tofu for added protein, and pack the bowl with a side of salsa or avocado for extra flavor.

3. **Egg and Vegetable Stir-Fry:** Sauté diced vegetables (such as bell peppers, broccoli, and snap peas) with scrambled eggs and cooked shrimp or tofu in a skillet. Season with soy sauce, garlic, and ginger for a flavorful and protein-rich stir-fry option.

4. **Turkey and Cheese Roll-Ups:** Roll slices of deli turkey or chicken breast around string cheese or sliced avocado for a quick and portable protein-packed lunch option. Add a side

of raw vegetables or almonds for added crunch and nutrition.

5. **Salmon and Avocado Sushi Bowl:** Combine cooked salmon, sliced avocado, cucumber strips, and seaweed salad in a bowl. Drizzle with soy sauce or tamari and sprinkle with sesame seeds for a satisfying and protein-rich sushi-inspired lunch option.

6. **Protein-Packed Salad Jars:** Layer cooked quinoa, chickpeas, diced vegetables, and grilled chicken or tofu in a mason jar. Top with mixed greens and your favorite dressing, and shake the jar before eating for a convenient and protein-packed lunch option.

7. **Greek Yogurt Parfait:** Layer Greek yogurt with mixed berries, nuts, and seeds in a portable container for a protein-rich and satisfying lunch option. Add a drizzle of honey or sugar-free syrup for sweetness, if desired.

8. **Tuna Salad Lettuce Wraps:** Mix canned tuna with mayonnaise, diced celery, red onion, and lemon juice. Spoon the tuna salad onto large lettuce leaves and roll up to create low carb wraps. Pack the wraps with a side of sliced vegetables or almonds for a satisfying and protein-packed lunch option.

9. **Protein-Packed Soup:** Prepare a hearty soup with lean protein sources like chicken, turkey, or beans. Add plenty of vegetables and season with herbs and spices for flavor. Pack the soup in a thermos for a warm and satisfying lunch on the go.

10. **Cheese and Veggie Skewers:** Thread cherry tomatoes, cucumber slices, and cubes of cheese onto skewers for a portable and protein-packed snack or lunch option. Pair the skewers with whole grain crackers or a piece of fruit for a balanced meal.

These protein-packed lunch ideas are perfect for maintaining energy levels and keeping you feeling satisfied throughout the day. Whether you prefer salads, wraps, or bowls, these options are easy to prepare and convenient for on-the-go eating.

Creative Low Carb Lunch Ideas for Work or School

When it comes to low carb lunches for work or school, creativity is key. Here are some creative and delicious low carb lunch ideas to keep you fueled throughout the day:

1. **Zucchini Noodle Salad:** Toss spiralized zucchini noodles with cherry tomatoes, olives, feta cheese, and Italian dressing for a refreshing and low carb salad option. Add grilled chicken or tofu for extra protein, if desired.

2. **Stuffed Bell Peppers:** Fill halved bell peppers with a mixture of ground turkey or beef, cooked quinoa, diced vegetables, and shredded cheese. Bake until tender for a flavorful and protein-rich lunch option.

3. **Cauliflower Fried Rice:** Sauté cauliflower rice with diced vegetables, scrambled eggs, and cooked shrimp or tofu in a skillet. Season with soy sauce, garlic, and ginger for a delicious and low carb twist on traditional fried rice.

4. **Eggplant Parmesan:** Bake sliced eggplant rounds with marinara sauce and shredded mozzarella cheese until bubbly and golden. Serve with a side salad for a satisfying and low carb lunch option.

5. **Turkey Lettuce Wraps:** Fill large lettuce leaves with sliced turkey breast, avocado slices, bacon strips, and tomato slices. Drizzle with mayonnaise or ranch dressing and roll up the lettuce leaves to create low carb wraps.

6. **Cucumber Subs:** Slice a cucumber in half lengthwise and hollow out the center to create a cucumber "sub." Fill the cucumber halves with deli meat, cheese slices, and your favorite sandwich toppings for a low carb twist on a classic sub sandwich.

7. **Spaghetti Squash Pad Thai:** Roast spaghetti squash strands and toss with cooked shrimp or tofu, bean sprouts, carrots,

and peanuts in a homemade pad Thai sauce. Garnish with lime wedges and cilantro for a flavorful and low carb lunch option.

8. **Mason Jar Salads:** Layer chopped vegetables, protein sources (such as grilled chicken, hard-boiled eggs, or chickpeas), and mixed greens in a mason jar. Top with your favorite dressing and shake the jar before eating for a convenient and portable lunch option.

9. **Low Carb Wraps:** Use low carb tortillas or lettuce leaves as wraps and fill with your favorite sandwich fillings, such as turkey, cheese, avocado, and bacon. Roll up the wraps and slice into pinwheels for a satisfying and portable lunch option.

10. **Sushi Bowls:** Prepare a sushi-inspired bowl with cauliflower rice, cooked shrimp or crab, avocado slices, cucumber strips, and seaweed salad. Drizzle with soy sauce or tamari and sprinkle with sesame seeds for a flavorful and low carb lunch option.

These creative low carb lunch ideas are perfect for work or school and are sure to keep you satisfied and fueled throughout the day. Whether you prefer salads, wraps, or bowls, these options are easy to prepare and packed with flavor.

CHAPTER FIVE

Flavorful Dinners Without the Carbs

One-Pan Meals for Simple and Low Carb Dinners

One-pan meals are perfect for busy weeknights when you want a delicious dinner without the hassle of multiple pots and pans. Here are some flavorful one-pan recipes that are low in carbs:

1. **Sheet Pan Lemon Herb Chicken:** Arrange chicken breasts on a sheet pan with sliced lemon, garlic cloves, and fresh herbs such as rosemary and thyme. Drizzle with olive oil and season with salt and pepper. Add your choice of low carb vegetables such as asparagus, broccoli, or Brussels sprouts to the pan. Roast in the oven until the chicken is cooked through and the vegetables are tender for a flavorful and easy dinner option.

2. **One-Pan Salmon and Asparagus:** Place salmon fillets on a sheet pan and surround them with trimmed asparagus spears. Drizzle with olive oil and season with salt, pepper, and lemon zest. Bake in the oven until the salmon is flaky and the asparagus is tender for a simple and nutritious dinner option.

3. **Cauliflower Fried Rice:** Sauté diced vegetables such as bell peppers, onions, and carrots in a large skillet until tender. Push the vegetables to one side of the skillet and add beaten eggs to the empty side. Scramble the eggs until cooked through, then stir to combine with the vegetables. Add riced cauliflower to the skillet and stir-fry until heated through. Season with soy sauce, garlic, and ginger for a flavorful and low carb twist on traditional fried rice.

4. **One-Pot Zucchini Noodle Primavera:** Sauté diced vegetables such as bell peppers, cherry tomatoes, and mushrooms in a large pot until tender. Add spiralized zucchini noodles to the pot and toss to combine with the vegetables. Stir in a jar of marinara sauce and simmer until heated through. Serve topped with grated Parmesan cheese for a quick and satisfying low carb dinner option.

5. **Skillet Garlic Butter Shrimp:** Sauté shrimp in a skillet with minced garlic, butter, and lemon juice until pink and opaque. Add chopped parsley and red pepper flakes for added flavor and heat. Serve the shrimp over sautéed spinach or cauliflower rice for a simple and flavorful low carb dinner option.

6. **Mexican Cauliflower Rice Skillet:** Cook ground turkey or beef in a skillet with diced onions and bell peppers until browned. Stir in riced cauliflower, diced tomatoes, and

Mexican-inspired seasonings such as chili powder, cumin, and paprika. Simmer until heated through and garnish with chopped cilantro and sliced avocado for a flavorful and satisfying low carb dinner option.

7. **Sheet Pan Sausage and Vegetable Bake:** Slice Italian sausage links and toss with diced vegetables such as bell peppers, onions, and zucchini on a sheet pan. Drizzle with olive oil and season with Italian seasoning, salt, and pepper. Roast in the oven until the sausage is browned and the vegetables are tender for an easy and flavorful low carb dinner option.

8. **One-Pan Lemon Garlic Butter Chicken Thighs:** Brown chicken thighs in a skillet with minced garlic and olive oil. Add chicken broth, lemon juice, and butter to the skillet and simmer until the chicken is cooked through and the sauce is reduced. Serve the chicken thighs with steamed green beans or broccoli for a simple and flavorful low carb dinner option.

9. **Sautéed Shrimp and Broccoli Stir-Fry:** Sauté shrimp in a skillet with minced garlic, ginger, and soy sauce until pink and opaque. Add broccoli florets to the skillet and stir-fry until tender-crisp. Serve the shrimp and broccoli over cauliflower rice for a quick and flavorful low carb dinner option.

10. **Sheet Pan Pork Chop and Vegetable Bake:** Season pork chops with your favorite spices and arrange them on a sheet

pan with diced sweet potatoes, Brussels sprouts, and red onion. Drizzle with olive oil and season with salt, pepper, and rosemary. Roast in the oven until the pork chops are cooked through and the vegetables are tender for a hearty and satisfying low carb dinner option.

These one-pan meals are perfect for simple and flavorful low carb dinners that require minimal cleanup. Experiment with different proteins, vegetables, and seasonings to create your own delicious combinations.

Vegetarian and Plant-Based Dinner Options

Following a low carb diet doesn't mean you have to skimp on flavor or variety, especially if you're vegetarian or looking to incorporate more plant-based meals into your diet. Here are some flavorful vegetarian and plant-based dinner options that are low in carbs:

1. **Cauliflower Crust Pizza:** Make a low carb pizza crust using cauliflower rice, almond flour, and eggs. Top the crust with marinara sauce, shredded cheese, and your favorite vegetable toppings such as sliced bell peppers, mushrooms, and olives. Bake until the crust is crispy and the cheese is melted for a delicious and low carb pizza option.

2. **Zucchini Noodle Alfredo:** Spiralize zucchini into noodles and sauté in a skillet with minced garlic and olive oil until tender. Toss the zucchini noodles with Alfredo sauce made from

heavy cream, Parmesan cheese, and garlic. Serve topped with chopped parsley and grated Parmesan cheese for a creamy and low carb pasta alternative.

3. **Eggplant Parmesan:** Slice eggplant into rounds and dip in beaten eggs, then coat with a mixture of almond flour, Parmesan cheese, and Italian seasonings. Bake until the eggplant is golden and crispy, then layer with marinara sauce and mozzarella cheese. Bake until bubbly and serve with a side of steamed vegetables for a satisfying and low carb dinner option.

4. **Portobello Mushroom Burgers:** Grill portobello mushroom caps until tender and juicy, then serve on low carb hamburger buns or lettuce wraps with your favorite burger toppings such as avocado slices, tomato slices, and red onion. Serve with a side of roasted vegetables or a salad for a flavorful and satisfying plant-based dinner option.

5. **Stuffed Bell Peppers:** Fill halved bell peppers with a mixture of cooked quinoa, black beans, diced tomatoes, and shredded cheese. Bake until the peppers are tender and the filling is heated through. Serve topped with salsa and sliced avocado for a flavorful and protein-rich vegetarian dinner option.

6. **Cauliflower Fried Rice:** Sauté diced vegetables such as bell peppers, onions, and carrots in a large skillet until tender.

Push the vegetables to one side of the skillet and add beaten eggs to the empty side. Scramble the eggs until cooked through, then stir to combine with the vegetables. Add riced cauliflower to the skillet and stir-fry until heated through. Season with soy sauce, garlic, and ginger for a flavorful and low carb twist on traditional fried rice.

7. **Stuffed Portobello Mushrooms:** Remove the stems from portobello mushrooms and fill the caps with a mixture of spinach, ricotta cheese, minced garlic, and Italian seasonings. Bake until the mushrooms are tender and the filling is heated through. Serve topped with marinara sauce and grated Parmesan cheese for a flavorful and low carb dinner option.

8. **Cauliflower Crust Veggie Flatbread:** Make a cauliflower crust using cauliflower rice, almond flour, and eggs, then shape into a flatbread shape. Top the crust with pesto sauce, sliced tomatoes, mozzarella cheese, and fresh basil. Bake until the crust is crispy and the cheese is melted for a delicious and low carb flatbread option.

9. **Vegetarian Stir-Fry:** Sauté diced tofu or tempeh in a skillet with minced garlic, ginger, and soy sauce until golden and crispy. Add diced vegetables such as bell peppers, broccoli, and snap peas to the skillet and stir-fry until tender-crisp.

Serve over cauliflower rice or shirataki noodles for a flavorful and low carb dinner option.

10.   **Zucchini Lasagna:** Slice zucchini into thin strips and layer in a baking dish with marinara sauce, ricotta cheese, and shredded mozzarella cheese. Repeat the layers until the dish is full, then bake until the cheese is melted and bubbly. Serve with a side salad for a satisfying and low carb twist on traditional lasagna.

These vegetarian and plant-based dinner options are flavorful and satisfying, making them perfect for those following a low carb lifestyle. Experiment with different ingredients and flavors to create your own delicious and nutritious plant-based meals.

Slow Cooker and Instant Pot Recipes for Effortless Low Carb Meals

Using a slow cooker or Instant Pot is a convenient way to prepare flavorful and low carb meals with minimal effort. Here are some delicious slow cooker and Instant Pot recipes that are perfect for busy weeknights:

Slow Cooker Recipes:

1. **Crockpot Chicken Taco Soup:** Combine diced chicken breasts, diced tomatoes, black beans, diced bell peppers, onions, and Mexican-inspired seasonings such as chili powder, cumin, and paprika in a slow cooker. Cook on low

for 6-8 hours or high for 3-4 hours until the chicken is cooked through and the flavors are melded together. Serve topped with shredded cheese, avocado slices, and fresh cilantro for a flavorful and low carb soup option.

2. **Slow Cooker Beef Stew:** Brown stew meat in a skillet and transfer to a slow cooker. Add diced carrots, celery, onions, and mushrooms to the slow cooker along with beef broth, tomato paste, and Italian seasonings. Cook on low for 6-8 hours or high for 3-4 hours until the beef is tender and the vegetables are cooked through. Serve hot for a hearty and low carb dinner option.

3. **Crockpot Pork Carnitas:** Season pork shoulder with Mexican-inspired spices such as cumin, chili powder, and oregano. Place the pork shoulder in a slow cooker with diced onions, minced garlic, and orange juice. Cook on low for 8-10 hours or high for 4-6 hours until the pork is tender and shreds easily with a fork. Serve the pork carnitas in lettuce wraps or over cauliflower rice with your favorite toppings such as salsa, guacamole, and diced onions for a flavorful and low carb dinner option.

4. **Slow Cooker Chicken Curry:** Combine diced chicken breasts, diced bell peppers, onions, coconut milk, and curry paste in a slow cooker. Cook on low for 6-8 hours or high for 3-4 hours until the chicken is cooked through and the flavors are

melded together. Serve over cauliflower rice for a flavorful and low carb curry option.

5. **Crockpot Chili:** Brown ground beef or turkey in a skillet and transfer to a slow cooker. Add diced tomatoes, tomato sauce, diced bell peppers, onions, garlic, chili powder, cumin, and paprika to the slow cooker. Cook on low for 6-8 hours or high for 3-4 hours until the flavors are melded together and the chili is thick and hearty. Serve topped with shredded cheese, sour cream, and sliced green onions for a delicious and low carb dinner option.

Instant Pot Recipes:

1. **Instant Pot Lemon Garlic Chicken:** Season chicken breasts with minced garlic, lemon zest, lemon juice, and Italian seasonings. Place the chicken breasts in the Instant Pot with chicken broth and cook on high pressure for 8 minutes. Quick release the pressure and remove the chicken from the Instant Pot. Stir in heavy cream and grated Parmesan cheese to make a creamy sauce. Serve the chicken with the sauce over cauliflower rice for a flavorful and low carb dinner option.

2. **Instant Pot Beef and Broccoli:** Brown sliced beef sirloin in the Instant Pot using the sauté function. Remove the beef from the Instant Pot and set aside. Add diced onions, minced garlic, soy sauce, beef broth, and ginger to the Instant Pot

and stir to combine. Return the beef to the Instant Pot along with broccoli florets and cook on high pressure for 5 minutes. Quick release the pressure and serve the beef and broccoli over cauliflower rice for a flavorful and low carb dinner option.

3. **Instant Pot Butter Chicken:** Sauté diced onions, minced garlic, ginger, and Indian-inspired spices such as garam masala, turmeric, and coriander in the Instant Pot using the sauté function. Add diced chicken breasts, diced tomatoes, tomato paste, and coconut milk to the Instant Pot and stir to combine. Cook on high pressure for 8 minutes, then natural release the pressure for 10 minutes. Stir in heavy cream and serve the butter chicken over cauliflower rice for a flavorful and low carb dinner option.

4. **Instant Pot Spaghetti Squash with Meatballs:** Cut a spaghetti squash in half lengthwise and remove the seeds. Place the squash halves in the Instant Pot with water and cook on high pressure for 10 minutes. Quick release the pressure and remove the squash from the Instant Pot. Use a fork to shred the squash into spaghetti-like strands. Serve the spaghetti squash with cooked meatballs and marinara sauce for a flavorful and low carb dinner option.

5. **Instant Pot Chicken and Vegetable Soup:** Combine diced chicken breasts, diced carrots, celery, onions, garlic, chicken

broth, Italian seasonings, and salt and pepper in the Instant Pot. Cook on high pressure for 8 minutes, then quick release the pressure. Stir in chopped spinach or kale and cook on the sauté function until wilted. Serve hot for a comforting and low carb dinner option.

These slow cooker and Instant Pot recipes are perfect for effortless low carb meals that are packed with flavor. Whether you prefer soups, stews, or curries, these options are sure to satisfy your cravings while keeping you on track with your low carb lifestyle.

CHAPTER SIX

Snacks to Keep Blood Sugar Stable

Nutritious Low Carb Snack Ideas for Between Meals

Maintaining stable blood sugar levels is crucial for overall health, especially for individuals managing conditions like diabetes. Here are some nutritious low carb snack ideas to keep blood sugar stable between meals:

1. **Cheese and Veggie Sticks:** Pair sliced cheese with crunchy vegetable sticks such as carrots, celery, and bell peppers for a satisfying and low carb snack option. The protein and fiber in this snack combo help keep you full and satisfied while stabilizing blood sugar levels.

2. **Hard-Boiled Eggs:** Hard-boiled eggs are an excellent source of protein and healthy fats, making them a perfect low carb snack to keep blood sugar stable. Enjoy them on their own or sprinkle with salt and pepper for extra flavor.

3. **Greek Yogurt with Berries:** Greek yogurt is high in protein and low in carbs, making it an ideal snack for stabilizing blood sugar levels. Top Greek yogurt with fresh berries such

as strawberries, blueberries, or raspberries for added sweetness and antioxidants.

4. **Nuts and Seeds:** Nuts and seeds are packed with protein, healthy fats, and fiber, making them a nutritious and low carb snack option. Enjoy a handful of almonds, walnuts, or pumpkin seeds for a satisfying snack that helps keep blood sugar stable.

5. **Avocado with Tomato Slices:** Avocado is rich in healthy fats and fiber, making it a great option for stabilizing blood sugar levels. Enjoy sliced avocado with tomato slices sprinkled with salt and pepper for a simple and nutritious low carb snack.

6. **Cottage Cheese with Cucumber Slices:** Cottage cheese is high in protein and low in carbs, making it an excellent snack choice for stabilizing blood sugar levels. Enjoy cottage cheese with cucumber slices for a refreshing and satisfying snack option.

7. **Celery with Peanut Butter:** Celery sticks filled with peanut butter are a classic low carb snack that's rich in protein, healthy fats, and fiber. Opt for natural peanut butter without added sugars for the healthiest option.

8. **Jerky:** Beef or turkey jerky is a convenient and portable snack that's high in protein and low in carbs, making it perfect for stabilizing blood sugar levels between meals.

Look for jerky options without added sugars or preservatives for the healthiest choice.

9. **Edamame:** Edamame, or steamed soybeans, is a nutritious and low carb snack option that's rich in protein and fiber. Enjoy edamame seasoned with sea salt for a satisfying and flavorful snack.

10. **Cucumber Slices with Tuna Salad:** Cucumber slices topped with tuna salad make a delicious and low carb snack that's packed with protein and healthy fats. Mix canned tuna with mayonnaise, diced celery, and lemon juice, then spoon onto cucumber slices for a tasty and satisfying snack option.

These nutritious low carb snack ideas are perfect for stabilizing blood sugar levels between meals while providing essential nutrients and keeping you feeling satisfied throughout the day.

Homemade Snacks That Are Low in Carbs and High in Flavor

When it comes to homemade snacks, you can create delicious and low carb options that are packed with flavor. Here are some homemade snack ideas that are low in carbs and high in flavor:

1. **Cauliflower Hummus with Veggie Sticks:** Make homemade hummus using cauliflower instead of chickpeas for a low carb twist on this classic snack. Pair the cauliflower hummus with crunchy vegetable sticks such as carrots, celery, and cucumber for a satisfying and flavorful snack option.

2. **Parmesan Crisps:** Bake grated Parmesan cheese on a parchment-lined baking sheet until crispy for a delicious and low carb snack that's packed with flavor. Enjoy Parmesan crisps on their own or pair them with sliced vegetables for dipping.

3. **Kale Chips:** Toss kale leaves with olive oil, salt, and your favorite seasonings such as garlic powder, paprika, or nutritional yeast. Bake the kale leaves in the oven until crispy for a flavorful and nutritious low carb snack option.

4. **Buffalo Cauliflower Bites:** Toss cauliflower florets with buffalo sauce and olive oil, then bake in the oven until crispy for a spicy and flavorful low carb snack. Serve the buffalo cauliflower bites with ranch dressing or blue cheese dip for dipping.

5. **Stuffed Mini Peppers:** Fill mini bell peppers with a mixture of cream cheese, shredded cheese, and chopped herbs such as chives or parsley for a flavorful and low carb snack option. Bake the stuffed peppers in the oven until the cheese is melted and bubbly for a delicious appetizer or snack.

6. **Spicy Roasted Chickpeas:** Toss cooked chickpeas with olive oil, smoked paprika, cayenne pepper, and sea salt. Roast the chickpeas in the oven until crispy for a spicy and flavorful low carb snack option.

7. **Zucchini Chips:** Slice zucchini into thin rounds and toss with olive oil, salt, and pepper. Bake the zucchini slices in the oven until crispy for a tasty and low carb snack option. Serve the zucchini chips with marinara sauce or ranch dressing for dipping.

8. **Eggplant Bruschetta:** Slice eggplant into rounds and grill or roast until tender. Top the eggplant rounds with diced tomatoes, minced garlic, fresh basil, and balsamic glaze for a flavorful and low carb snack option.

9. **Coconut Almond Energy Bites:** Combine almond flour, shredded coconut, almond butter, honey or a low carb sweetener, and vanilla extract in a bowl. Roll the mixture into bite-sized balls and refrigerate until firm for a delicious and satisfying snack option.

10. **Cucumber Sushi Rolls:** Use cucumber slices as a low carb alternative to sushi rice and roll with your favorite sushi fillings such as avocado, cucumber, smoked salmon, or crab for a flavorful and nutritious snack option.

These homemade snack ideas are perfect for satisfying your cravings while keeping you on track with your low carb lifestyle. Experiment with different flavors and ingredients to create your own delicious and nutritious snacks at home.

Portable Snacks for On-the-Go Convenience

When you're on the go, having portable snacks on hand is essential for keeping blood sugar stable and avoiding unhealthy temptations. Here are some portable snack ideas that are low in carbs and perfect for on-the-go convenience:

1. **String Cheese:** String cheese is a convenient and portable snack that's low in carbs and high in protein, making it perfect for on-the-go convenience. Enjoy string cheese on its own or pair it with sliced vegetables or nuts for added flavor and nutrition.

2. **Beef Jerky:** Beef jerky is a convenient and portable snack that's high in protein and low in carbs, making it perfect for on-the-go convenience. Look for beef jerky options without added sugars or preservatives for the healthiest choice.

3. **Nut Butter Packets:** Individual packets of nut butter such as almond butter or peanut butter are convenient and portable snacks that are low in carbs and high in protein and healthy fats. Enjoy nut butter packets on their own or pair them with sliced apples or celery sticks for a satisfying snack option.

4. **Seaweed Snacks:** Seaweed snacks are a convenient and portable snack option that's low in carbs and packed with essential nutrients such as vitamins, minerals, and antioxidants. Enjoy seaweed snacks on their own or pair

them with sliced avocado for a flavorful and nutritious snack option.

5. **Protein Bars:** Protein bars are a convenient and portable snack option that's low in carbs and high in protein, making them perfect for on-the-go convenience. Look for protein bars with minimal added sugars and ingredients for the healthiest choice.

6. **Boiled Eggs:** Hard-boiled eggs are a convenient and portable snack option that's low in carbs and high in protein, making them perfect for on-the-go convenience. Enjoy boiled eggs on their own or pair them with sliced vegetables or cheese for added flavor and nutrition.

7. **Cheese Crisps:** Cheese crisps are a convenient and portable snack option that's low in carbs and packed with flavor. Enjoy cheese crisps on their own or pair them with sliced vegetables or deli meat for added flavor and nutrition.

8. **Roasted Chickpeas:** Roasted chickpeas are a convenient and portable snack option that's low in carbs and packed with protein and fiber. Enjoy roasted chickpeas on their own or pair them with sliced vegetables or nuts for added flavor and nutrition.

9. **Trail Mix:** Trail mix is a convenient and portable snack option that's low in carbs and packed with protein, healthy fats, and

fiber. Look for trail mix options with minimal added sugars and ingredients for the healthiest choice.

10.   **Sliced Vegetables with Dip:** Sliced vegetables such as carrots, celery, and bell peppers are a convenient and portable snack option that's low in carbs and packed with essential nutrients. Pair sliced vegetables with your favorite dip such as hummus or guacamole for added flavor and nutrition.

These portable snack ideas are perfect for on-the-go convenience and can help keep blood sugar stable while providing essential nutrients and keeping you feeling satisfied throughout the day. Keep these snacks on hand for busy days when you need a quick and convenient option to keep you fueled and energized.

CHAPTER SEVEN

Satisfying Low Carb Desserts

Lower Carb Dessert Recipes for Sweet Cravings

Satisfying your sweet tooth while maintaining a low carb lifestyle is entirely possible with the right recipes. Here are some lower carb dessert recipes that are sure to satisfy your sweet cravings without derailing your diet:

1. **Keto Cheesecake:** This creamy and indulgent dessert is made with a low carb almond flour crust and a rich filling of cream cheese, eggs, and sweetened with a low carb sweetener like erythritol or stevia. Top with a sugar-free berry compote for extra flavor.

2. **Chocolate Avocado Mousse:** Avocado adds creaminess to this decadent chocolate mousse while keeping it low in carbs and high in healthy fats. Blend ripe avocados with unsweetened cocoa powder, almond milk, and your choice of low carb sweetener until smooth and creamy. Chill before serving for the perfect texture.

3. **Low Carb Peanut Butter Cookies:** These chewy and satisfying cookies are made with almond flour, natural peanut butter, and a low carb sweetener. With just a few simple ingredients, you can enjoy a delicious sweet treat without the guilt.

4. **Coconut Flour Pancakes:** Pancakes aren't just for breakfast! These fluffy and flavorful pancakes made with coconut flour are perfect for a low carb dessert. Top with sugar-free syrup or whipped cream for added sweetness.

5. **Sugar-Free Chocolate Bark:** Melt dark chocolate (70% cocoa or higher) and spread it thinly on a baking sheet lined with parchment paper. Sprinkle with chopped nuts, coconut flakes, or sea salt for extra flavor and crunch. Once set, break into pieces and enjoy as a satisfying low carb dessert.

6. **Low Carb Lemon Bars:** These tangy and refreshing lemon bars are made with a buttery almond flour crust and a zesty lemon filling sweetened with a low carb sweetener. Dust with powdered erythritol for a finishing touch.

7. **Chia Seed Pudding:** Chia seeds are packed with fiber and healthy fats, making them a great ingredient for a low carb dessert. Mix chia seeds with unsweetened almond milk and your choice of low carb sweetener, then let it sit in the fridge overnight to thicken. Top with fresh berries or nuts before serving.

8. **Almond Flour Brownies:** These rich and fudgy brownies are made with almond flour, cocoa powder, eggs, and a low carb sweetener. They're a perfect indulgence for when you're craving something sweet but want to keep it low carb.

9. **Low Carb Berry Crisp:** This fruity dessert is made with a mix of fresh berries such as strawberries, blueberries, and raspberries, topped with a crumbly mixture of almond flour, butter, and a low carb sweetener. Bake until golden and bubbly for a delicious and satisfying treat.

10. **Sugar-Free Popsicles:** Blend together your favorite low carb fruits such as berries, citrus, or melon with water or coconut water and a low carb sweetener. Pour the mixture into popsicle molds and freeze until solid for a refreshing and guilt-free dessert option.

These lower carb dessert recipes are perfect for satisfying your sweet cravings while keeping you on track with your low carb lifestyle. Experiment with different flavors and ingredients to create your own delicious and satisfying sweet treats.

Fruit-Based Desserts That Are Naturally Low in Carbs

Fruit-based desserts can be a delicious and naturally low carb option for satisfying your sweet tooth. Here are some fruit-based dessert ideas that are perfect for those following a low carb lifestyle:

1. **Berries with Whipped Cream:** Fresh berries such as strawberries, raspberries, and blueberries are naturally low in carbs and packed with antioxidants. Serve them with a dollop of homemade whipped cream made with heavy cream and a low carb sweetener for a simple and satisfying dessert option.

2. **Grilled Peaches with Cinnamon:** Grilling peaches brings out their natural sweetness and caramelizes their sugars, making them a delicious and low carb dessert option. Sprinkle grilled peaches with cinnamon and serve with a scoop of sugar-free vanilla ice cream for a decadent treat.

3. **Chia Seed Fruit Parfait:** Layer fresh berries with chia seed pudding made with unsweetened almond milk and a low carb sweetener for a delicious and nutritious dessert option. Top with chopped nuts or shredded coconut for added texture and flavor.

4. **Baked Apples with Cinnamon:** Baked apples are a comforting and low carb dessert option that's perfect for fall. Core apples and fill them with a mixture of cinnamon, nutmeg, and a low carb sweetener. Bake until tender and serve warm with a drizzle of sugar-free caramel sauce for extra indulgence.

5. **Coconut Lime Popsicles:** Blend together coconut milk, lime juice, and a low carb sweetener until smooth. Pour the mixture into popsicle molds and freeze until solid for a refreshing and tropical dessert option that's low in carbs.

6. **Chocolate-Dipped Strawberries:** Dip fresh strawberries in melted dark chocolate (70% cocoa or higher) and place them on a parchment-lined baking sheet. Chill in the fridge until the chocolate is set for a simple and elegant low carb dessert option.

7. **Watermelon Mint Salad:** Cube watermelon and toss with fresh mint leaves for a refreshing and low carb dessert option that's perfect for summer. Serve chilled for extra refreshment.

8. **Kiwi Sorbet:** Blend peeled kiwi fruit with a squeeze of lime juice and a low carb sweetener until smooth. Freeze the mixture in an ice cream maker according to the manufacturer's instructions for a refreshing and low carb sorbet option.

9. **Mixed Berry Compote:** Simmer fresh or frozen berries with a splash of water and a low carb sweetener until they break down and form a thick sauce. Serve warm or chilled over Greek yogurt or low carb pancakes for a satisfying and fruity dessert option.

10.   **Cantaloupe with Prosciutto:** Wrap thin slices of prosciutto around cubes of ripe cantaloupe for a sweet and savory low carb dessert option that's perfect for entertaining.

These fruit-based dessert ideas are perfect for satisfying your sweet cravings while keeping you on track with your low carb lifestyle. Enjoy them as a healthy and delicious way to indulge in something sweet without the guilt.

Indulgent Treats Made Healthier with Low Carb Ingredients

Indulging in your favorite treats doesn't have to derail your low carb lifestyle. With a few simple swaps, you can enjoy all the flavors you love while keeping it low carb. Here are some indulgent treats made healthier with low carb ingredients:

1. **Keto Chocolate Chip Cookies:** These chewy and satisfying cookies are made with almond flour, sugar-free chocolate chips, and a low carb sweetener. With just a few simple swaps, you can enjoy all the flavors of your favorite chocolate chip cookies without the guilt.

2. **Low Carb Ice Cream:** There are plenty of low carb ice cream options available on the market, or you can make your own at home using ingredients like coconut milk, heavy cream, and a low carb sweetener. Add in your favorite mix-ins such

as nuts, chocolate chips, or fruit for a delicious and indulgent treat.

3. **Avocado Chocolate Pudding:** Avocado adds creaminess to this rich and decadent chocolate pudding while keeping it low in carbs and high in healthy fats. Blend ripe avocados with cocoa powder, almond milk, and a low carb sweetener until smooth and creamy for a guilt-free indulgence.

4. **Low Carb Brownie Bites:** These bite-sized brownies are made with almond flour, unsweetened cocoa powder, eggs, and a low carb sweetener. They're perfect for satisfying your chocolate cravings without derailing your low carb lifestyle.

5. **Chocolate Covered Strawberries:** Dip fresh strawberries in melted dark chocolate (70% cocoa or higher) and chill until the chocolate is set for a decadent and indulgent treat that's low in carbs. Enjoy them as a sweet and satisfying dessert option.

6. **Low Carb Cheesecake Bars:** These creamy and indulgent cheesecake bars are made with a low carb almond flour crust and a rich filling of cream cheese, eggs, and a low carb sweetener. Top with sugar-free fruit compote or whipped cream for extra flavor.

7. **Peanut Butter Cup Fat Bombs:** These bite-sized treats are made with a mixture of natural peanut butter, coconut oil,

and a low carb sweetener. They're perfect for satisfying your sweet cravings while providing a boost of healthy fats.

8. **Chocolate Avocado Truffles:** These rich and creamy truffles are made with avocado, cocoa powder, coconut oil, and a low carb sweetener. Roll the mixture into balls and coat with chopped nuts or shredded coconut for a delicious and indulgent treat.

9. **Low Carb Chocolate Cake:** This moist and decadent chocolate cake is made with almond flour, cocoa powder, eggs, and a low carb sweetener. Top with sugar-free chocolate ganache or whipped cream for extra indulgence.

10. **Salted Caramel Cheesecake Fat Bombs:** These bite-sized treats are made with a mixture of cream cheese, butter, caramel extract, and a low carb sweetener. They're perfect for satisfying your sweet cravings while providing a boost of healthy fats.

These indulgent treats made healthier with low carb ingredients are perfect for satisfying your sweet cravings while keeping you on track with your low carb lifestyle. Enjoy them as a guilt-free way to indulge in your favorite flavors without derailing your diet.

CHAPTER EIGHT

Side Dishes to Accompany Any Meal

Simple and Delicious Vegetable Side Dishes

Vegetable side dishes are not only nutritious but also versatile and delicious. Here are some simple and delicious vegetable side dishes that can accompany any meal:

1. **Roasted Vegetables:** Toss a variety of vegetables such as carrots, broccoli, cauliflower, Brussels sprouts, and bell peppers with olive oil, salt, pepper, and your favorite herbs or spices. Roast in the oven until tender and caramelized for a flavorful and nutritious side dish.

2. **Sautéed Greens:** Sauté leafy greens such as spinach, kale, or Swiss chard with garlic and olive oil until wilted. Season with salt, pepper, and a squeeze of lemon juice for a simple and nutritious side dish.

3. **Stir-Fried Vegetables:** Stir-fry a mix of colorful vegetables such as bell peppers, snap peas, carrots, and mushrooms in a hot skillet with sesame oil and soy sauce until crisp-tender. Garnish with sesame seeds and green onions for added flavor.

4. **Grilled Asparagus:** Toss asparagus spears with olive oil, salt, and pepper, then grill until tender and lightly charred for a delicious and elegant side dish.

5. **Cauliflower Mash:** Steam or boil cauliflower florets until tender, then mash with butter, garlic, and your choice of herbs or spices for a low carb alternative to mashed potatoes.

6. **Zucchini Noodles (Zoodles):** Use a spiralizer to create zucchini noodles, then sauté them in a hot skillet with olive oil and garlic until tender. Serve as a light and refreshing alternative to pasta.

7. **Green Bean Almondine:** Blanch green beans in boiling water until crisp-tender, then sauté with sliced almonds, butter, and lemon zest for a flavorful and elegant side dish.

8. **Cucumber Salad:** Thinly slice cucumbers and toss with red onion, cherry tomatoes, feta cheese, olive oil, and balsamic vinegar for a refreshing and colorful side dish.

9. **Brussels Sprouts Slaw:** Shred Brussels sprouts and toss with shredded carrots, sliced apples, dried cranberries, and a creamy dressing for a crunchy and flavorful side dish.

10. **Eggplant Caponata:** Sauté diced eggplant with onions, garlic, tomatoes, olives, capers, and vinegar until soft and flavorful for a Mediterranean-inspired side dish.

These simple and delicious vegetable side dishes are perfect for accompanying any meal and adding color, flavor, and nutrients to your plate.

Low Carb Grain and Legume Alternatives for Sides

If you're looking for low carb alternatives to grains and legumes, there are plenty of options to choose from. Here are some low carb grain and legume alternatives for sides that are nutritious and delicious:

1. **Cauliflower Rice:** Pulse cauliflower florets in a food processor until they resemble rice grains, then sauté in a hot skillet with olive oil and garlic until tender for a low carb alternative to rice.

2. **Broccoli Rice:** Follow the same process as cauliflower rice, but use broccoli florets instead for a nutritious and flavorful low carb alternative to rice.

3. **Spaghetti Squash:** Roast or microwave spaghetti squash until tender, then scrape the flesh with a fork to create spaghetti-like strands for a low carb alternative to pasta.

4. **Shirataki Noodles:** These noodles are made from konjac yam and are extremely low in carbs and calories. Simply rinse and drain them well, then cook in a hot skillet with your favorite sauce or toppings for a low carb alternative to traditional noodles.

5. **Zucchini Lasagna:** Use thinly sliced zucchini in place of lasagna noodles in your favorite lasagna recipe for a low carb alternative that's just as satisfying and delicious.

6. **Cabbage Wraps:** Use blanched cabbage leaves as a wrapper for fillings such as ground meat, rice, and vegetables for a low carb alternative to tortillas or wraps.

7. **Portobello Mushroom Caps:** Use grilled or roasted portobello mushroom caps as a base for pizza toppings, burger patties, or sandwiches for a low carb alternative to bread or crusts.

8. **Cauliflower Mash:** Steam or boil cauliflower florets until tender, then mash with butter, cream, and your choice of herbs or spices for a low carb alternative to mashed potatoes.

9. **Lettuce Wraps:** Use large lettuce leaves such as iceberg or romaine as a wrapper for fillings such as grilled chicken, shrimp, or tofu for a low carb alternative to tacos or sandwiches.

10. **Cucumber Slices:** Use thinly sliced cucumber rounds as a base for toppings such as smoked salmon, cream cheese, and dill for a low carb alternative to crackers or bread.

These low carb grain and legume alternatives for sides are perfect for adding variety and nutrition to your meals while keeping your carb intake in check.

Creative Ways to Add Flavor to Your Low Carb Side Dishes

Adding flavor to your low carb side dishes doesn't have to mean adding extra carbs. Here are some creative ways to enhance the flavor of your low carb side dishes without sacrificing taste:

1. **Herb Butter:** Make a compound butter by mixing softened butter with chopped fresh herbs such as parsley, basil, or thyme. Spread over steamed vegetables or grilled meats for a burst of flavor.

2. **Lemon Zest:** Grate lemon zest over roasted vegetables or sautéed greens for a bright and citrusy flavor that complements their natural sweetness.

3. **Garlic and Onion:** Sauté minced garlic and onion in olive oil until golden and fragrant, then toss with cooked vegetables or stir into cauliflower rice for added depth of flavor.

4. **Toasted Nuts:** Toast chopped nuts such as almonds, walnuts, or pine nuts in a dry skillet until golden and fragrant, then sprinkle over salads or vegetable dishes for added crunch and flavor.

5. **Fresh Herbs:** Chop fresh herbs such as parsley, cilantro, or dill and sprinkle over cooked vegetables or salads for a burst of freshness and flavor.

6. **Parmesan Cheese:** Grate Parmesan cheese over roasted vegetables or cauliflower rice for a nutty and savory flavor that enhances their natural sweetness.

7. **Balsamic Glaze:** Drizzle balsamic glaze over grilled vegetables or caprese salad for a tangy and sweet flavor that adds depth to the dish.

8. **Hot Sauce:** Add a splash of hot sauce or chili paste to sautéed vegetables or cauliflower rice for a spicy kick that wakes up the taste buds.

9. **Soy Sauce or Tamari:** Stir-fry vegetables with soy sauce or tamari for a savory and umami-rich flavor that pairs well with grilled meats or tofu.

10. **Coconut Milk:** Add coconut milk to cauliflower rice or curried vegetables for a creamy and tropical flavor that adds richness to the dish.

These creative ways to add flavor to your low carb side dishes are perfect for enhancing their taste without adding extra carbs. Experiment with different ingredients and combinations to find your favorite flavor combinations.

CHAPTER NINE

Dining Out and Socializing with Diabetes

Eating out and socializing can present challenges for individuals managing diabetes, but with the right strategies and communication techniques, it's possible to enjoy these occasions while still prioritizing your health.

Strategies for Eating Low Carb When Dining Out

Dining out doesn't have to derail your low carb diet or blood sugar management. Here are some strategies for eating low carb when dining out:

1. **Research the Menu in Advance:** Many restaurants offer their menus online, allowing you to review the options and plan your meal ahead of time. Look for dishes that are naturally low in carbs or can be easily modified to fit your dietary needs.

2. **Choose Protein and Vegetable-Based Dishes:**Opt for dishes that are centered around lean protein sources such as grilled chicken, fish, or steak, paired with non-starchy vegetables like salad greens, broccoli, or asparagus. These options are typically lower in carbs and higher in nutrients.

3. **Ask for Modifications:** Don't be afraid to ask your server for modifications to accommodate your low carb diet. Request

substitutions such as extra vegetables instead of rice or potatoes, or ask for sauces and dressings on the side to control your carb intake.

4. **Avoid Bread and Appetizers:** Skip the bread basket and appetizers like breaded or fried items, which are typically high in carbs. Instead, focus on the main course and choose options that align with your dietary goals.

5. **Be Mindful of Hidden Carbs:** Pay attention to hidden sources of carbs in sauces, marinades, and condiments. Ask your server about the ingredients used in dishes and choose options that are prepared without added sugars or starchy thickeners.

6. **Portion Control:** Restaurant portions tend to be larger than what you might eat at home, so consider splitting an entree with a dining companion or asking for a half portion to avoid overeating.

7. **Stick to Water or Unsweetened Beverages:** Avoid sugary drinks like soda, juice, or cocktails, which can quickly spike blood sugar levels. Opt for water, unsweetened iced tea, or sparkling water with a splash of lemon or lime instead.

8. **Don't Skip Dessert, but Choose Wisely:** If you're craving something sweet, look for low carb dessert options like berries with whipped cream, a cheese plate, or a small

square of dark chocolate. Remember to enjoy these treats in moderation.

9. **Practice Portion Awareness:** Pay attention to portion sizes and consider using visual cues like the size of your palm or a deck of cards to gauge appropriate serving sizes. This can help you avoid overeating and keep your carb intake in check.

10. **Stay Flexible and Forgiving:** If you end up eating something higher in carbs than you planned, don't dwell on it. Focus on making the best choices you can in the moment and move on. One meal or snack won't derail your progress as long as you get back on track with your next choice.

By following these strategies, you can enjoy dining out while still adhering to your low carb diet and managing your diabetes effectively.

Tips for Navigating Social Events and Special Occasions

Social events and special occasions often revolve around food, which can present challenges for individuals managing diabetes. Here are some tips for navigating these situations:

1. **Plan Ahead:** If you know you'll be attending a social event or special occasion, plan your meals and snacks for the day accordingly. Eat a balanced meal with protein, healthy fats,

and fiber before the event to help stabilize your blood sugar levels.

2. **Bring Your Own Dish:** Offer to bring a low carb dish or appetizer to share at social gatherings. This ensures that you'll have something healthy and diabetes-friendly to enjoy while also introducing others to delicious low carb options.

3. **Focus on Socializing, Not Just Food:** While food is often a central part of social events, remember that the primary purpose is to connect with others and enjoy their company. Focus on engaging in conversation and activities rather than solely on the food.

4. **Be Selective with Your Choices:** Scan the buffet or appetizer table and choose items that align with your dietary goals. Fill your plate with protein-rich foods like grilled chicken or shrimp, along with non-starchy vegetables like salad greens or crudites.

5. **Watch Your Alcohol Intake:** Alcohol can affect blood sugar levels and may interfere with diabetes management, especially if consumed in excess. If you choose to drink, opt for lower carb options like dry wine, light beer, or spirits mixed with club soda or seltzer.

6. **Practice Portion Control:** Be mindful of portion sizes and avoid going back for seconds unless you're truly hungry. Use

smaller plates and utensils to help control your portions and prevent overeating.

7. **Stay Hydrated:** Drink plenty of water throughout the event to stay hydrated and help prevent overeating. Sometimes thirst can be mistaken for hunger, so staying hydrated can help curb unnecessary snacking.

8. **Manage Stress and Anxiety:** Social events can sometimes be stressful or anxiety-provoking, which may lead to emotional eating or unhealthy food choices. Practice stress management techniques such as deep breathing, mindfulness, or talking to a supportive friend or family member.

9. **Be Prepared to Educate Others:** Be prepared to educate friends and family members about your dietary needs and why you're making certain food choices. Use these opportunities as teaching moments to raise awareness and promote understanding about diabetes and low carb eating.

10. **Give Yourself Grace:** Remember that it's okay to indulge occasionally and enjoy special treats in moderation. Don't beat yourself up if you veer off track slightly during social events or special occasions. Focus on making the best choices you can in the moment and move forward with your diabetes management plan.

By following these tips, you can navigate social events and special occasions with confidence while still prioritizing your health and managing your diabetes effectively.

How to Communicate Your Dietary Needs Effectively

Effective communication is key when it comes to dining out or attending social events with diabetes. Here are some tips for communicating your dietary needs effectively:

1. **Be Clear and Specific:** Clearly communicate your dietary needs and preferences to restaurant staff or hosts when dining out or attending social events. Use specific language and provide details about what you can and cannot eat.

2. **Ask Questions:** Don't be afraid to ask questions about menu items or how dishes are prepared. Inquire about ingredients, cooking methods, and possible substitutions to ensure that your meal meets your dietary requirements.

3. **Use "I" Statements:** When discussing your dietary needs with others, use "I" statements to express your preferences and concerns without placing blame or making others feel defensive. For example, say, "I need to avoid high carb foods to manage my diabetes" rather than "You can't serve me that."

4. **Provide Solutions:** Offer suggestions or alternatives when communicating your dietary needs to restaurant staff or

hosts. For example, say, "Could I substitute steamed vegetables for the rice?" or "Would it be possible to have the sauce on the side?"

5. **Be Assertive, Not Aggressive:** Assertively communicate your dietary needs without being confrontational or aggressive. Approach the conversation with a positive and collaborative attitude, and be willing to work together to find solutions that meet everyone's needs.

6. **Express Gratitude:** Show appreciation to restaurant staff or hosts for accommodating your dietary needs and for their willingness to make modifications or provide alternatives. A simple "thank you" goes a long way in fostering positive communication.

7. **Follow Up if Necessary:** If you have specific dietary restrictions or concerns, consider following up with restaurant staff or hosts in advance to ensure that your needs will be met. This extra step can help prevent misunderstandings and ensure a positive dining experience.

8. **Educate Others:** Take the opportunity to educate friends, family members, and restaurant staff about diabetes and low carb eating. Share information about your dietary needs and the reasons behind your food choices to promote understanding and awareness.

9. **Stay Calm and Patient:** Remain calm and patient if there are misunderstandings or challenges when communicating your dietary needs. Remember that most people want to be helpful and accommodating, but may not fully understand the complexities of managing diabetes.

10.   **Advocate for Yourself:** Advocate for yourself and your dietary needs with confidence and assertiveness. Your health and well-being are important, and it's okay to speak up and ensure that your needs are met when dining out or socializing.

By following these tips, you can effectively communicate your dietary needs and preferences while dining out or attending social events with diabetes, ensuring that you can enjoy these occasions while still prioritizing your health and well-being.

CHAPTER TEN

Meal Planning and Prep for Low Carb Success

Practical Tips for Low Carb Meal Planning and Grocery Shopping

Meal planning and grocery shopping are essential components of a successful low carb lifestyle. Here are some practical tips to help you plan and shop for low carb meals effectively:

1. **Start with a Plan:** Before you head to the grocery store, take some time to plan your meals for the week. Look for low carb recipes that you enjoy and create a meal plan that includes a variety of protein sources, vegetables, and healthy fats.

2. **Make a List:** Once you have your meal plan in place, make a list of the ingredients you'll need for each recipe. Organize your list by category (e.g., produce, dairy, protein) to make shopping more efficient and ensure you don't forget anything.

3. **Shop the Perimeter:** When navigating the grocery store, focus on the perimeter where you'll find fresh produce, meats, dairy, and other whole foods. This is where you'll find the majority of low carb options, while processed and high carb foods are typically located in the center aisles.

4. **Choose Whole Foods:**Opt for whole, minimally processed foods whenever possible. Fresh fruits and vegetables, lean meats, poultry, fish, eggs, nuts, seeds, and healthy fats like avocado and olive oil should form the foundation of your low carb diet.

5. **Read Labels Carefully:** When selecting packaged foods, be sure to read the nutrition labels carefully. Look for products that are low in carbs and free from added sugars, refined grains, and unhealthy fats. Pay attention to serving sizes to avoid hidden carbs.

6. **Stock Up on Staples:** Keep your pantry stocked with low carb staples such as almond flour, coconut flour, coconut oil, olive oil, herbs, spices, and sugar-free condiments like mustard, hot sauce, and salsa. Having these ingredients on hand makes it easier to whip up low carb meals on the fly.

7. **Choose Frozen and Canned Options:** Don't overlook frozen and canned options, which can be just as nutritious as fresh and are often more budget-friendly. Look for frozen vegetables, berries, and seafood, as well as canned meats, beans, and tomatoes with no added sugars or sauces.

8. **Shop Seasonally:** Take advantage of seasonal produce, which tends to be fresher, more flavorful, and often more affordable. Visit farmers' markets or join a CSA (Community

Supported Agriculture) to access locally grown, seasonal fruits and vegetables.

9. **Be Flexible:** While it's important to stick to your meal plan and grocery list as much as possible, be flexible and open to making substitutions if needed. If a certain ingredient isn't available or is too expensive, look for alternatives that fit within your low carb goals.

10. **Avoid Shopping Hungry:** Shopping on an empty stomach can lead to impulse purchases of high carb, processed foods. Eat a balanced meal or snack before heading to the grocery store to help curb cravings and make healthier choices.

By following these practical tips for low carb meal planning and grocery shopping, you can set yourself up for success and make it easier to stick to your low carb lifestyle.

Batch Cooking and Freezing Low Carb Meals for Convenience

Batch cooking and freezing meals in advance can save you time and effort while ensuring that you always have healthy low carb options on hand. Here are some strategies for batch cooking and freezing low carb meals for convenience:

1. **Choose Freezer-Friendly Recipes:** Look for recipes that freeze well and maintain their taste and texture after

thawing. Casseroles, soups, stews, chili, and meatballs are all excellent options for batch cooking and freezing.

2. **Invest in Quality Containers:** Invest in high-quality freezer-safe containers and storage bags to keep your meals fresh and prevent freezer burn. Choose containers that are BPA-free and can be easily labeled with the date and contents.

3. **Label and Date Everything:** Label each container or bag with the name of the dish and the date it was prepared. This makes it easy to identify what's in the freezer and how long it's been there, helping you avoid food waste.

4. **Portion Meals Appropriately:** Portion your meals into individual or family-sized servings before freezing to make mealtime prep a breeze. This allows you to thaw and reheat only what you need, reducing waste and ensuring you always have the right portion size.

5. **Cool Foods Properly:** Allow cooked foods to cool to room temperature before transferring them to the freezer to prevent condensation and ice crystals from forming. Once cooled, cover and refrigerate the dishes for a few hours before transferring them to the freezer for long-term storage.

6. **Use Proper Thawing Techniques:** When it's time to enjoy your frozen meals, thaw them safely in the refrigerator

overnight or use the defrost setting on your microwave for faster thawing. Avoid thawing at room temperature, as this can promote bacterial growth.

7. **Reheat Safely:** Reheat frozen meals thoroughly to an internal temperature of 165°F (74°C) to ensure they are safe to eat. Use a microwave, oven, stovetop, or slow cooker to reheat dishes evenly, stirring occasionally if needed.

8. **Rotate Your Stock:** Keep track of what's in your freezer and rotate your stock regularly to ensure you're using up older meals first. This helps prevent food waste and ensures that your meals are always fresh and delicious.

9. **Experiment with New Recipes:** Use batch cooking as an opportunity to experiment with new low carb recipes and flavors. Get creative with ingredients and spices to keep your meals interesting and satisfying.

10. **Enjoy the Convenience:** Embrace the convenience of batch cooking and freezing meals, knowing that you always have healthy low carb options available, even on your busiest days. Enjoy the extra time and peace of mind that comes with having meals ready to go whenever you need them.

By incorporating batch cooking and freezing into your meal prep routine, you can save time, reduce stress, and maintain a healthy low carb diet with ease.

Strategies for Portion Control and Balanced Low Carb Eating

Portion control is an important aspect of balanced low carb eating, helping you manage your calorie intake and maintain a healthy weight. Here are some strategies for portion control and balanced low carb eating:

1. **Use Smaller Plates:**Opt for smaller plates and bowls to help control portion sizes. Research shows that using smaller dishes can trick your brain into feeling more satisfied with smaller portions.

2. **Fill Half Your Plate with Vegetables:** Aim to fill half of your plate with non-starchy vegetables such as leafy greens, broccoli, cauliflower, zucchini, and bell peppers. These foods are low in carbs and calories but high in fiber, vitamins, and minerals, helping you feel full and satisfied.

3. **Portion Protein Properly:** Include a moderate portion of protein with each meal, such as chicken, fish, tofu, or lean beef. Aim for a serving size that's about the size of your palm or a deck of cards, which is roughly 3-4 ounces for most people.

4. **Limit Starchy Foods:** While some starchy foods like potatoes, rice, and grains can be part of a balanced diet, it's important to watch your portion sizes, especially if you're following a low carb eating plan. Opt for smaller servings or choose low carb alternatives like cauliflower rice or spiralized vegetables.

5. **Measure Portions:** Use measuring cups, spoons, or a food scale to accurately measure portions of foods like grains, nuts, seeds, and high carb vegetables. This can help prevent overeating and ensure that you're sticking to your low carb goals.

6. **Practice Mindful Eating:** Pay attention to your hunger and fullness cues while eating, and stop when you feel satisfied rather than overly full. Eating slowly, savoring each bite, and chewing thoroughly can help you tune into your body's signals and prevent overeating.

7. **Plan Balanced Meals:** Aim for balanced meals that include a combination of protein, healthy fats, and fiber-rich carbohydrates. This helps keep you feeling full and satisfied while providing your body with the nutrients it needs for optimal health.

8. **Snack Wisely:** Choose nutrient-dense, low carb snacks like nuts, seeds, cheese, Greek yogurt, or sliced vegetables with

hummus. Portion out snacks in advance to prevent mindless munching and help control your calorie intake.

9. **Stay Hydrated:** Drink plenty of water throughout the day to stay hydrated and help control hunger. Sometimes thirst can be mistaken for hunger, so staying hydrated can help prevent overeating.

10. **Listen to Your Body:** Pay attention to how different foods make you feel and adjust your portion sizes accordingly. If you find that certain foods spike your blood sugar or leave you feeling sluggish, consider reducing your portion sizes or avoiding those foods altogether.

By incorporating these strategies into your daily routine, you can practice portion control and maintain a balanced low carb diet that supports your health and well-being.

Meal planning and prep are essential for maintaining a successful low carb lifestyle. By following these practical tips for meal planning and grocery shopping, batch cooking and freezing low carb meals, and practicing portion control and balanced eating, you can enjoy delicious and nutritious meals while managing your diabetes effectively. With careful planning and preparation, you can set yourself up for long-term success and make low carb living a sustainable and enjoyable lifestyle choice.

SparkPeople Diet:

Definition:

The SparkPeople Diet is an online weight loss and wellness program that offers tools, resources, and support for individuals looking to achieve their health and fitness goals. The program provides personalized meal plans, workout routines, tracking tools, and a supportive community to help participants make sustainable lifestyle changes. The SparkPeople Diet focuses on a balanced approach to nutrition, exercise, and behavior change, emphasizing portion control, mindful eating, and regular physical activity. It encourages participants to set realistic goals, track progress, and celebrate successes along the way.

Ingredients:

- Balanced Meals: SparkPeople provides personalized meal plans tailored to individual dietary preferences, calorie needs, and weight loss goals.

- Nutrient-Dense Foods: Participants are encouraged to incorporate a variety of fruits, vegetables, whole grains, lean proteins, and healthy fats into their meals and snacks.

- Portion Control: SparkPeople emphasizes portion control techniques such as measuring food portions, using smaller plates, and being mindful of serving sizes to manage calorie intake.

- Exercise Routines: SparkPeople offers workout routines and fitness videos for participants to incorporate regular physical activity into their daily routines.

- Tracking Tools: SparkPeople provides tracking tools for food intake, exercise, weight loss progress, and other health metrics to help participants stay accountable and monitor their success.

- Supportive Community: SparkPeople offers a supportive online community where participants can connect with others, share experiences, and receive encouragement and motivation.

Instructions/How to Prepare:

1. Sign up for the SparkPeople program and create a personalized profile, including information about dietary preferences, weight loss goals, and activity level.

2. Receive personalized meal plans, workout routines, and tracking tools based on individual needs and goals.

3. Follow the SparkPeople meal plan, incorporating a variety of nutrient-dense foods such as fruits, vegetables, whole grains, lean proteins, and healthy fats into meals and snacks.

4. Practice portion control by measuring food portions, using smaller plates, and being mindful of serving sizes to manage calorie intake.

5. Incorporate regular physical activity into daily routines, following SparkPeople workout routines and fitness videos or engaging in other forms of exercise that are enjoyable and sustainable.

6. Use SparkPeople tracking tools to monitor food intake, exercise, weight loss progress, and other health metrics, staying accountable and motivated along the way.

7. Engage with the SparkPeople community, connecting with others, sharing experiences, and receiving encouragement and support throughout the weight loss journey.

8. Be patient and consistent, recognizing that weight loss and lifestyle changes take time and effort, and celebrating successes along the way.

9. Adjust meal plans, workout routines, and goals as needed based on progress and feedback, staying flexible and adaptable to individual needs and preferences.

10.   Embrace a lifelong commitment to health and wellness, incorporating healthy habits into daily life and continuing to strive for improvement and success.

The Insulin-Resistance Diet:

Definition:

The Insulin-Resistance Diet is a dietary approach aimed at managing insulin resistance, a condition in which cells become less responsive to the effects of insulin, leading to elevated blood sugar levels. This diet focuses on regulating blood sugar levels, improving insulin sensitivity, and promoting overall health and well-being. It emphasizes whole, nutrient-dense foods that have a minimal impact on blood sugar levels, such as non-starchy vegetables, lean proteins, healthy fats, and high-fiber carbohydrates. The Insulin-Resistance Diet also encourages regular physical activity, stress management, and lifestyle modifications to support metabolic health.

Ingredients:

- Whole Foods: Non-starchy vegetables, leafy greens, lean proteins, nuts, seeds, legumes, whole grains, healthy fats, and low-glycemic fruits are emphasized on The Insulin-Resistance Diet.

- High-Fiber Carbohydrates: Carbohydrates with a high fiber content, such as whole grains, legumes, fruits, and vegetables, are preferred to support stable blood sugar levels and promote satiety.

- Lean Proteins: Lean sources of protein, including poultry, fish, tofu, tempeh, legumes, and low-fat dairy products, are prioritized to support muscle health and metabolic function.

- Healthy Fats: Monounsaturated and polyunsaturated fats from sources such as avocados, nuts, seeds, olive oil, and fatty fish are encouraged to provide essential nutrients and support cardiovascular health.

- Low-Glycemic Foods: Foods with a low glycemic index, which have a minimal impact on blood sugar levels, are favored on The Insulin-Resistance Diet to help regulate insulin levels and prevent spikes and crashes in blood sugar.

Instructions/How to Prepare:

1. Educate yourself about insulin resistance and how dietary and lifestyle factors can influence blood sugar levels and insulin sensitivity.

2. Stock your kitchen with whole, nutrient-dense foods such as non-starchy vegetables, leafy greens, lean proteins, nuts, seeds, legumes, whole grains, healthy fats, and low-glycemic fruits.

3. Plan meals and snacks that prioritize whole foods and balance macronutrients to support stable blood sugar levels and improve insulin sensitivity.

4. Focus on eating a variety of colors, flavors, and textures in meals to ensure a diverse intake of nutrients and promote satiety and enjoyment.

5. Choose high-fiber carbohydrates such as whole grains, legumes, fruits, and vegetables to slow the absorption of sugar into the bloodstream and prevent spikes in blood sugar levels.

6. Incorporate lean sources of protein into meals and snacks to support muscle health, promote satiety, and stabilize blood sugar levels.

7. Include healthy fats from sources such as avocados, nuts, seeds, olive oil, and fatty fish to provide essential nutrients and support cardiovascular health.

8. Minimize or eliminate processed foods, refined sugars, artificial additives, trans fats, and other inflammatory substances from your diet to reduce inflammation and improve metabolic health.

9. Pay attention to portion sizes and practice mindful eating by listening to hunger and fullness cues, eating slowly, and savoring each bite.

10. Stay hydrated by drinking plenty of water throughout the day to support overall health and well-being.

CHAPTER 11

DIET FOR DIABETES

Mediterranean Diet:

Definition:

The Mediterranean diet is inspired by the traditional dietary patterns of countries bordering the Mediterranean Sea. It emphasizes whole, minimally processed foods such as fruits, vegetables, whole grains, nuts, seeds, legumes, fish, and olive oil. It limits red meat and sweets, while encouraging moderate consumption of dairy products, poultry, and eggs.

Ingredients:

- Fruits: Berries, apples, oranges, grapes, etc.

- Vegetables: Spinach, tomatoes, peppers, onions, etc.

- Whole Grains: Whole wheat bread, brown rice, quinoa, oats, etc.

- Nuts and Seeds: Almonds, walnuts, flaxseeds, chia seeds, etc.

- Legumes: Chickpeas, lentils, beans, etc.

- Fish and Seafood: Salmon, tuna, shrimp, etc.

- Olive Oil: Extra virgin olive oil for cooking and dressing.

- Herbs and Spices: Basil, oregano, garlic, cumin, etc.

Instructions/How to Prepare:

1. Base meals around plant-based foods like fruits, vegetables, whole grains, and legumes.

2. Use olive oil as the primary source of fat for cooking and dressing salads.

3. Incorporate fish and seafood into your diet regularly, aiming for at least two servings per week.

4. Enjoy moderate amounts of poultry, eggs, and dairy products, such as yogurt and cheese.

5. Limit red meat consumption to a few times per month.

6. Snack on nuts and seeds for a healthy source of fats and protein.

7. Flavor meals with herbs and spices instead of salt.

8. Drink plenty of water and enjoy a moderate amount of red wine if desired (optional).

DASH Diet (Dietary Approaches to Stop Hypertension):

Definition:

The DASH diet is specifically designed to help lower blood pressure and reduce the risk of hypertension. It emphasizes fruits, vegetables, whole grains, and lean proteins while limiting sodium, saturated fats, and sweets.

Ingredients:

- Fruits: Berries, bananas, apples, oranges, etc.

- Vegetables: Leafy greens, carrots, broccoli, bell peppers, etc.

- Whole Grains: Brown rice, whole wheat bread, quinoa, oats, barley, etc.

- Lean Proteins: Chicken breast, turkey, fish, tofu, beans, lentils, etc.

- Dairy: Low-fat or fat-free milk, yogurt, cheese, etc.

- Nuts and Seeds: Almonds, pistachios, sunflower seeds, etc.

- Healthy Fats: Olive oil, avocado, nuts, seeds, etc.

Instructions/How to Prepare:

1. Focus on incorporating plenty of fruits and vegetables into your meals and snacks.

2. Choose whole grains over refined grains whenever possible.

3. Opt for lean proteins such as poultry, fish, tofu, and legumes.

4. Limit high-fat dairy products and opt for low-fat or fat-free options.

5. Include nuts and seeds as snacks or in salads for added nutrients and healthy fats.

6. Use herbs, spices, and citrus juices to flavor foods instead of salt.

7. Avoid processed and high-sodium foods like canned soups, packaged snacks, and fast food.

8. Cook meals at home whenever possible to have better control over ingredients and portion sizes.

9. Aim to limit sweets and sugary beverages, opting for natural sweeteners like fruit when craving something sweet.

10. Stay hydrated by drinking plenty of water throughout the day.

Low-Carb Diet:

Definition:

A low-carb diet involves reducing carbohydrate intake while increasing the consumption of protein and healthy fats. This diet aims to control insulin levels, promote weight loss, and improve overall health by limiting foods high in carbohydrates such as bread, pasta, rice, and sugary snacks.

Ingredients:

- Protein Sources: Meat, poultry, fish, tofu, tempeh, eggs.

- Non-Starchy Vegetables: Leafy greens, broccoli, cauliflower, zucchini, bell peppers.

- Healthy Fats: Avocado, nuts, seeds, olive oil, coconut oil.

- Dairy: Cheese, Greek yogurt, cottage cheese (in moderation).

- Low-Carb Fruits: Berries, avocados, tomatoes, lemons, limes.

- Herbs and Spices: Basil, oregano, garlic, turmeric, cumin.

- Sweeteners (optional): Stevia, erythritol, monk fruit.

Instructions/How to Prepare:

1. Focus on whole, unprocessed foods.

2. Limit carbohydrate intake to around 20-50 grams per day, depending on individual needs and goals.

3. Include protein-rich foods in each meal to promote satiety and muscle maintenance.

4. Fill up on non-starchy vegetables to increase fiber intake and provide essential vitamins and minerals.

5. Incorporate healthy fats into your diet for energy and to keep you feeling full.

6. Be mindful of hidden carbs in sauces, condiments, and processed foods.

7. Drink plenty of water to stay hydrated and support overall health.

8. Experiment with low-carb recipes and meal prep to make adhering to the diet easier and more enjoyable.

Ketogenic Diet (Keto Diet):

Definition:

The ketogenic diet is a very low-carb, high-fat diet that forces the body to enter a state of ketosis, where it primarily burns fat for fuel instead of carbohydrates. This diet has been used for decades to treat epilepsy and has gained popularity for weight loss and improving metabolic health.

Ingredients:

- Healthy Fats: Avocado, coconut oil, olive oil, butter, ghee, fatty fish.

- Protein Sources: Meat, poultry, fish, eggs, tofu, tempeh.

- Non-Starchy Vegetables: Leafy greens, broccoli, cauliflower, zucchini, asparagus.

- Full-Fat Dairy: Cheese, heavy cream, Greek yogurt (in moderation).

- Nuts and Seeds: Macadamia nuts, almonds, chia seeds, flaxseeds.

- Low-Carb Fruits: Berries (in moderation), avocado.

- Herbs and Spices: Turmeric, ginger, cinnamon, garlic, thyme.

- Sweeteners (in moderation): Stevia, erythritol, monk fruit.

Instructions/How to Prepare:

1. Keep carbohydrate intake extremely low, typically below 20-50 grams per day to induce and maintain ketosis.

2. Consume moderate amounts of protein, as excessive protein intake can potentially hinder ketosis.

3. Base meals around healthy fats, such as avocados, olive oil, and fatty fish.

4. Incorporate non-starchy vegetables to provide essential nutrients and fiber while keeping carbohydrate intake low.

5. Be mindful of hidden carbs in foods and beverages, including sauces, dressings, and flavored beverages.

6. Stay hydrated by drinking plenty of water, as dehydration can occur more easily on a ketogenic diet.

7. Monitor ketone levels using urine strips, blood tests, or breath meters if desired, to ensure you are in ketosis.

8. Experiment with keto-friendly recipes and meal planning to maintain variety and enjoyment while following the diet.

The Sugar Busters Diet:

Definition:

The Sugar Busters Diet is a low-glycemic approach to eating that aims to control blood sugar levels and promote weight loss by minimizing the consumption of high-glycemic carbohydrates and sugars. It emphasizes whole, nutrient-dense foods that have a minimal impact on blood sugar levels, such as non-starchy vegetables, lean proteins, healthy fats, and low-glycemic carbohydrates. The Sugar Busters Diet also encourages portion control, regular physical activity, and lifestyle modifications to support metabolic health and overall well-being.

Ingredients:

- Whole Foods: Non-starchy vegetables, leafy greens, lean proteins, nuts, seeds, legumes, whole grains, healthy fats, and low-glycemic fruits are emphasized on The Sugar Busters Diet.

- Low-Glycemic Carbohydrates: Carbohydrates with a low glycemic index, such as whole grains, legumes, fruits, and vegetables, are preferred to help regulate blood sugar levels and prevent spikes and crashes in blood sugar.

- Lean Proteins: Lean sources of protein, including poultry, fish, tofu, tempeh, legumes, and low-fat dairy products, are prioritized to support muscle health and metabolic function.

- Healthy Fats: Monounsaturated and polyunsaturated fats from sources such as avocados, nuts, seeds, olive oil, and fatty fish are encouraged to provide essential nutrients and support cardiovascular health.

Instructions/How to Prepare:

1. Familiarize yourself with the principles of The Sugar Busters Diet, including recommendations for food choices, portion sizes, meal timing, and lifestyle habits.

2. Stock your kitchen with whole, nutrient-dense foods such as non-starchy vegetables, leafy greens, lean proteins, nuts, seeds, legumes, whole grains, healthy fats, and low-glycemic fruits.

3. Plan meals and snacks that prioritize whole foods and balance macronutrients to support stable blood sugar levels and improve insulin sensitivity.

4. Focus on eating a variety of colors, flavors, and textures in meals to ensure a diverse intake of nutrients and promote satiety and enjoyment.

5. Choose low-glycemic carbohydrates such as whole grains, legumes, fruits, and vegetables to help regulate blood sugar levels and prevent spikes and crashes in blood sugar.

6. Incorporate lean sources of protein into meals and snacks to support muscle health, promote satiety, and stabilize blood sugar levels.

7. Include healthy fats from sources such as avocados, nuts, seeds, olive oil, and fatty fish to provide essential nutrients and support cardiovascular health.

8. Practice portion control by measuring food portions, using smaller plates, and being mindful of serving sizes to manage calorie intake and support weight loss.

9. Stay hydrated by drinking plenty of water throughout the day to support overall health and well-being.

10. Incorporate regular physical activity into your daily routine to enhance metabolic function, support weight management, and promote overall fitness and well-being.

Here's a 31-day meal plan based on easy low-carb recipes from a diabetic cookbook for those newly diagnosed:

CHAPTER 12

31 DAYS MEAL PLAN

Week 1:

Day 1:

- Breakfast: Scrambled eggs with spinach and mushrooms.

- Lunch: Grilled chicken salad with mixed greens and avocado.

- Dinner: Baked salmon with roasted asparagus.

Day 2:

- Breakfast: Greek yogurt with raspberries and a sprinkle of chia seeds.

- Lunch: Turkey and cheese lettuce wraps with mustard.

- Dinner: Zucchini noodles with marinara sauce and grilled shrimp.

Day 3:

- Breakfast: Veggie omelette with bell peppers, onions, and cheese.

- Lunch: Tuna salad with cucumber slices.

- Dinner: Grilled steak with cauliflower mash.

Day 4:

- Breakfast: Smoothie with almond milk, spinach, and protein powder.

- Lunch: Egg salad with celery sticks.

- Dinner: Baked chicken thighs with broccoli florets.

Day 5:

- Breakfast: Cottage cheese with sliced strawberries and a drizzle of honey.

- Lunch: Caprese salad with tomato, mozzarella, and basil.

- Dinner: Stir-fried tofu with mixed vegetables.

Week 2:

Day 6:

- Breakfast: Scrambled eggs with spinach and feta cheese.

- Lunch: Turkey and cheese roll-ups with lettuce and mayonnaise.

- Dinner: Baked cod with lemon and herbs, served with sautéed spinach.

Day 7:

- Breakfast: Greek yogurt with blueberries and almonds.

- Lunch: Chicken Caesar salad with homemade dressing.

- Dinner: Beef stir-fry with bell peppers and broccoli.

Day 8:

- Breakfast: Chia seed pudding with unsweetened almond milk and sliced almonds.

- Lunch: Turkey avocado wrap with lettuce and tomato.

- Dinner: Grilled salmon with roasted Brussels sprouts.

Day 9:

- Breakfast: Veggie scramble with tomatoes, onions, and mushrooms.

- Lunch: Cobb salad with grilled chicken, bacon, avocado, and hard-boiled egg.

- Dinner: Zucchini noodles with pesto and grilled shrimp.

Day 10:

- Breakfast: Smoothie bowl with mixed berries, spinach, and coconut flakes.

- Lunch: Tuna and avocado salad with mixed greens.

- Dinner: Baked chicken breast with steamed broccoli.

Week 3:

Day 11:

- Breakfast: Greek yogurt with sliced peaches and a sprinkle of cinnamon.

- Lunch: Turkey and cheese lettuce wraps with sliced bell peppers.

- Dinner: Grilled steak with roasted cauliflower.

Day 12:

- Breakfast: Scrambled eggs with spinach and tomatoes.

- Lunch: Chicken and avocado salad with balsamic vinaigrette.

- Dinner: Baked cod with sautéed zucchini.

Day 13:

- Breakfast: Cottage cheese with pineapple chunks and a sprinkle of cinnamon.

- Lunch: Greek salad with feta cheese, olives, and cucumbers.

- Dinner: Stir-fried tofu with broccoli and cauliflower rice.

Day 14:

- Breakfast: Omelette with bell peppers, onions, and cheese.

- Lunch: Turkey and cheese roll-ups with lettuce and mustard.

- Dinner: Grilled shrimp skewers with mixed greens salad.

Day 15:

- Breakfast: Smoothie with almond milk, strawberries, and protein powder.

- Lunch: Egg salad with celery sticks.

- Dinner: Baked chicken thighs with roasted asparagus.

Week 4:

Day 16:

- Breakfast: Greek yogurt with raspberries and a sprinkle of chia seeds.

- Lunch: Turkey avocado wrap with lettuce and tomato.

- Dinner: Grilled salmon with sautéed spinach.

Day 17:

- Breakfast: Scrambled eggs with spinach and feta cheese.

- Lunch: Cobb salad with grilled chicken, bacon, avocado, and hard-boiled egg.

- Dinner: Beef stir-fry with bell peppers and broccoli.

Day 18:

- Breakfast: Chia seed pudding with unsweetened almond milk and sliced almonds.

- Lunch: Tuna and avocado salad with mixed greens.

- Dinner: Baked chicken breast with steamed broccoli.

Day 19:

- Breakfast: Veggie scramble with tomatoes, onions, and mushrooms.
- Lunch: Turkey and cheese lettuce wraps with sliced bell peppers.
- Dinner: Grilled steak with roasted cauliflower.

Day 20:

- Breakfast: Smoothie bowl with mixed berries, spinach, and coconut flakes.
- Lunch: Greek salad with feta cheese, olives, and cucumbers.
- Dinner: Stir-fried tofu with broccoli and cauliflower rice.

Week 5:

Day 21:

- Breakfast: Cottage cheese with pineapple chunks and a sprinkle of cinnamon.
- Lunch: Turkey avocado wrap with lettuce and tomato.
- Dinner: Grilled shrimp skewers with mixed greens salad.

Day 22:

- Breakfast: Greek yogurt with raspberries and a sprinkle of chia seeds.

- Lunch: Egg salad with celery sticks.

- Dinner: Baked cod with sautéed zucchini.

Day 23:

- Breakfast: Scrambled eggs with spinach and tomatoes.

- Lunch: Chicken and avocado salad with balsamic vinaigrette.

- Dinner: Beef stir-fry with bell peppers and broccoli.

Day 24:

- Breakfast: Omelette with bell peppers, onions, and cheese.

- Lunch: Turkey and cheese roll-ups with lettuce and mustard.

- Dinner: Grilled salmon with sautéed spinach.

Day 25:

- Breakfast: Smoothie with almond milk, strawberries, and protein powder.

- Lunch: Cobb salad with grilled chicken, bacon, avocado, and hard-boiled egg.

- Dinner: Baked chicken thighs with roasted asparagus.

Week 6:

Day 26:

- Breakfast: Chia seed pudding with unsweetened almond milk and sliced almonds.

- Lunch: Tuna and avocado salad with mixed greens.

- Dinner: Grilled steak with roasted cauliflower.

Day 27:

- Breakfast: Veggie scramble with tomatoes, onions, and mushrooms.

- Lunch: Turkey and cheese lettuce wraps with sliced bell peppers.

- Dinner: Grilled shrimp skewers with mixed greens salad.

Day 28:

- Breakfast: Greek yogurt with raspberries and a sprinkle of chia seeds.

- Lunch: Egg salad with celery sticks.

- Dinner: Baked cod with sautéed zucchini.

Day 29:

- Breakfast: Scrambled eggs with spinach and feta cheese.

- Lunch: Chicken and avocado salad with balsamic vinaigrette.

- Dinner: Beef stir-fry with bell peppers and broccoli.

Day 30:

- Breakfast: Cottage cheese with pineapple chunks and a sprinkle of cinnamon.

- Lunch: Greek salad with feta cheese, olives, and cucumbers.

- Dinner: Stir-fried tofu with broccoli and cauliflower rice.

Day 31:

- Breakfast: Smoothie with almond milk, strawberries, and protein powder.

- Lunch: Turkey avocado wrap with lettuce and tomato.

- Dinner: Grilled salmon with sautéed spinach.

THE END